FANTASTIC VOYAGE III

Bernie Unrau DDS

CalTex Press

PO Box 69014
162 Ave S.W.
Calgary AB T2Y4S0
www.caltexpress.com

Published by Cal Tex Press
3413 16320 24 St SW
Calgary AB T2Y5A1
403-246-0523
www.caltexpress.com

ISBN 978-0-9866245-0-6

Printed by Amazon in San Bernardino, CA, US; Monee, IL, US; Fort Worth, TX, US; Philadelphia, PA, US; Columbia, SC, US; Mississauga, Ontario, CA; Leipzig, DE, EU; Luton, UK, EU; Torino, IT, EU; Narita, Chiba, JP; Wrocław, Poland, EU
https://www.amazon.com/-/e/B081M9Y1J9

FANTASTIC VOYAGE III c2010

1) Way To A Man's Heart
2) Trick or Treat?
3) Secrets
4) Take the Plunge
5) Gruesome
6) Fill 'er Up
7) Play Ball!
8) Message
9) Rocket to Russia?
10) Heart of the Matter
11) Beat of a Different Drum
12) Take a Stab at It
13) The Buck Stops Here!
14) Out of Sight?

PROLOGUE

Plagued with irreparable damage to his heart, president Taylor faced his worst fears. Two strikes to his name, the medical specialists placed his chances of survival at slim to nil. Having undergone coronary artery bypass graft surgery and artificial stent replacement before, his only hope now rested in the hands of the spirited nuclear submersible Proteus' crew and that of the medical specialists aboard. To attempt the world's first cardiac stem cell replacement therapy, that would hopefully jump start and rejuvenate the patient's ailing heart muscle. The weight of the world was upon his shoulders and those of the crew, those who had reluctantly signed onto the secret covert operation. Some even questioned the sanity of the scientists who had briefed them prior to departure. Reduced to the size of mere nanobots then injected into the blood stream in a race, to the heart, sufficient to boggle any one's mind. The brave crew knew the inherent risks. Like all the other races to be the first, the inner space race, no less spirited or challenging. This is their story.

1) Way To A Man's Heart

'The way to a man's heart is through his stomach…just make sure you thrust up through the ribcage.'

- Stephen Colbert, American political satirist, writer, TV host

The main lights were dimmed. The stainless steel surfaces muted from the hustle and bustle only a few hours ago. A solitary figure crept through the still silent room like a patient during an out of body experience following a fateful operation. The trim dapper culinary dilettante loosened the small bow tie affixed around his neck then undid the top button to his silk shirt, the black and white tuxedo still freshly pressed. The silhouette of a man then breathed a sigh of relief as if the weight of the world had been lifted off his shoulders or he'd passed through the pearly gates, parking himself in a pizzeria. A towering figure emerged from the shadows wielding a massive shiny stainless cleaver. The surgeon with no name raised the knife as if to make the final fateful incision. His odd tall chef's hat gave away his disguise, sworn to service and secrecy, the man swiftly sliced the multi tiered culinary creation in two. A few slices of fresh salad drizzled with a special secret dressing, fell from inside. The thick stacked layers of bacon, a host of deli delights and tomatoes parted easily. One could not ascertain the extent of how much high cholesterol or deleterious decadence saturated the sandwich.

"There you are mr president. The way to a man's heart is through his stomach….." he stated, always aiming to please. "..just make sure you thrust up through the ribcage" he added softly. He hoped the appetizer would provide the pick me up the distraught delegate deserved. His late night binging fests caused him some concern though. He'd been packing the carbs and calories on needlessly. Neither a physiologist nor or physical fitness instructor, he knew the leader of the free world was heading down a slippery slope to another heart attack. His condition had improved radically after the Whitehouse decided to grow a select line of organically grown omega three fatty acid embellished radishes and a host of garden variety of vegetables.

Try as he might, the president always aimed to please his audience, loyal campaign contributors and all the other world leaders. Desperate times demanded desperate measures he'd harped since the latest string of international incidents. The nuclear non proliferation talks, a million domestic distractions; why he was lucky he'd survived the ensuing issues and onslaught of paparazzi and White House reporters.

"Thanks James, that hit the spot" he stated savoring his decadent deli delight. The bountiful BLT variant barely fit into his gaping oral edifice.

The enticing herbs and spices tickled his palate. "I got a lot off my chest" he said, eager to savor and take another sumptuous bite. Over the monumental hurdle, the dicey state address, the rest of his term entered the home stretch. He was a shoe in for a second term reelection. Suddenly overcome by heart burning deep inside his chest, he grew dizzy, nauseous, disoriented. A pain shot up through his arm that encompassed his entire chest cavity. As if his kids or wife were sitting on his chest during a festive family outing at the farm. No, it was much worse, as if he'd been kicked by a raging bull. He dropped his sandwich and clutched his chest. His face dropped onto the plate piled sky high that mitigated the force of the impact in lieu of onto the cold stainless surface. His body slumped and slowly slid off the barstool at the opposite side of the table as the white house chef, James Callahan. It hit the cold tile floor without a flinch from the adept aging athlete. The body lay limp, lifeless, there in the darkness for a few seconds before the chef grasped the gravity of the gesture.

"Mr president?" The curious chef slowly

approached the prostrate body, then without a second thought tossed his chef's hat over his head across the room. He went down on the president, pounding his chest repeatedly in deliberate hard thumps, or CPR compressions, to the exquisite synchrony of an egg timer. Suddenly, a sign of life, refreshing but not out of the woods yet, he reached for the house phone to call 91 and an ambulance STAT! The secret service in situ sprung into action immediately. They'd rehearsed and planned for this scenario multiple times. The contingency plan in place, EMS and secret service attendants swiftly sent the prostrate body, pinned to a stretcher through a prearranged route through the under ground labyrinth to a waiting ambulance. The president was then whisked across town to a secret undisclosed underground facility near Bethesda Naval Hospital. The conspicuously cordoned off entrance was cluttered with security force, national guard and naval officers for a few moments as they awaited their commander in chief. An ominous silence fell upon Bethesda and the somber surrounding landscape. A light drizzle sprinkled the officers in full military attire, many coming home from a mixer at the Academy. It certainly put a damper on the department's award's dinner. Rumors circulated in the ensuing confusion. In a surreal dream like sequence an ambulance pulled up under a protective canopy. The patient was wheeled out from the back of the vehicle. EMS and secret service swarmed all around the president who was then hurried into the safe medical haven far below the streets of the capitol. Only a few of the officers sensed something was wrong, slightly intoxicated from the evening's entertainment and enticing cocktails. They caught a glimpse of their commander in chief. It happened so fast as EMS hurriedly applied several tubes, TPA infusers, monitors and lines as if stuffing the thanksgiving turkey. They stood speechless, their arms frozen at their sides rather than raising them in a stiff salute. The secret service donning their head sets, scoping out and securing the perimeter, scrambled to hustle the high ranking government official inside. The officers still stood in disbelief as the presidential seal surfaced several times before he went under cover of the canopy, then disappeared inside the sanctuary. President Taylor's dark distraught complexion, smiled faintly, heavily sedated, he slowly slipped into slumber. Losing control of his conscious and mental faculties, he wondered if this was the final curtain call. Immersed in images of his lovely first lady and children by his side. Even his trusty schnauzer, Scooter appeared and lapped at his face as the scrub nurse wiped the tasty treats from his cheeks and nose, the cause for the hallucination in his heavily sedated state. The attending veteran cardio thoracic surgeon on call began to deliberate and discuss their options as EMS presented the patient, a black male 50 in his prime political years. Vitals weak but stable, MI, myocardial infarction, a leading cause of death amongst middle aged, highly stressed type A personalities. Citing Circulation, a leading journal of the AMA- American Heart Association and countless other reputable reports, the precious seconds ticked by. The surgeon assessed and weighed his options and formulated his 'plan of attack'.

"Strike three?" questioned the ER staff. His medical history was promptly displayed on the robotic 'resident', now a permanent fixture in the hallowed halls. Out running, out reading, out prescribing the other physicians by the narrowest of margins. Even when at bat, most of the generals still preferred human touch and intervention to these latest medical advances and inventions. Yet his history of CHD, Coronary Heart Disease, soon mitigated and nullified several special delivery options.

"Too early to tell." They'd caught him in time, the TPA, the relentless clot buster beat its way through the barrage of blockages in his arteries, like Babe Ruth up to bat. He'd sent most balls out of the park and cleared the bases relentlessly. His past performances no less surprising. President Taylor had survived CABG, Coronary Artery Bypass Grafts, and Angioplasty twice before. The preliminary blood work and Chem 7 analysis compounded the problem. The prognosis didn't look promising.

The entourage decided to make their move. The trauma staff rushed the patient from the ER into a long hallway. They stopped outside a heavily fortified entrance. The retinal scanners positively ID'ed the men, as it rapidly ran an irritating beam of light across the back of their eyes like burning a DVD. Their fore finger print encrypted into the code cleared them. A final swipe of an unassuming card that looked like an Amex type credit card with bonus points for travel and eating out at any number of fine dining establishments hadn't crossed their minds. The specialists focused on the task at hand. To bring the patient back alive in the few fleeting minutes that remained.

In a noisy bar in downtown DC, a special news flash interrupted the regular broadcasting, a rerun of a Nationals hockey game, their imminent elimination bothered the dedicated hockey fans. Yet with all the other sports teams and distractions in DC, the Fox reporter soon took center stage outstanding in his field, in the rainy side streets of the capitol.

"The president's being rushed to Bethesda naval hospital for his 'routine annual physical'," he stated; it was all the press secretary released at this time. Even he wasn't convinced trying to pry anything from the staff, like using the jaws of life to extract a trapped toddler inside a sinking car in the Potomac. He raised the microphone to the press secretary leaving the White House in a hurry. "Excuse me, any word on the president's state of health?" he asked, all eyes glued to the overhead television screen. The fate of the free world, stock exchanges, financial institutions resting on his every word.

"The word is still mum, but just to let you in on a little secret" he stated reaffirmingly. The reporter's eyes lit up, as he wiped the condensation form his glasses. All eyes glued to their TV sets. "He's in the best hands, he'll undergo the most thorough exam by the best naval surgeons. He's in very good hands."

"He hasn't suffered another debilitating heart attack as was initially suspected?" asking point blank. With a sullen poker face, the press secretary repelled the catastrophic and untimely insinuation.

"No, definitely not," he said deceptively. "He's in the best of health. Why I'll bet he'll be up and at' em (atom?) in no time. "

"Care to place a wager on that?"

"Why, I'd bet my life on it." Why the political posturing albeit promising, the eternal optimist up to bat. The perfect pitch for a perplexed public.

The staff and specialists placed his chances at less than optimal. In fact his life now hung in the balance. Damocles' sword dangling over his life line, his golden chord. Nearer the end of the line and 60 minutes elapsed time. The press secretary swayed to side with more promising theoretical albeit oft untested palliative measures.

"There you have it. Just a routine procedure for president Taylor. God speed and God bless America." What the cunning press secretary hadn't impinged upon were similar circumstances during Grover Cleveland's term as president. On a more memorable outing he was quickly whisked aboard E.C. Benedict's yacht, the Oneida suffering from a slight 'tooth ache'. The surgery was performed by Dr Bryant, a New York dentist off Long Island right then and there on the bar's marble counter top much to the chagrin of the staff. The incident was dispelled and downplayed, a dramatic attempt to cover his cancerous growth, and eventual demise to the debilitating disease, suffering a fatal heart attack in 1908. The only president to serve two non consecutive terms, his last words were: 'I have tried so hard to do right.'

hexagonal box, like worker bees. Underneath the acronym CMDF, bold, large and clearly displayed.
Combined Miniaturization Deterrent Forces. Certainly a mouthful. No mention of it outside this select circle of colleagues or idle gossip and chatter at a capitol cocktail mixer.

The scene suddenly shifted to a tropical isle somewhere in the south pacific. The president's life flashing before his eyes? A beautiful round behind just out of reach from his lounger, in the small constricted field of vision, a spyglass? Bending over to reach a beach ball by the surfside. From the object of his obsession and delight, the tables were turned to a one full of cocktails adorned with tropical garnishes. The secret admirer peering through the aperture in a slice of cucumber, of his Pims #1 fruit flavored gin thirst quencher. We peered from his perspective out to the endless ocean. A sudden ringing in his ear drum, emanated across the sleepy stretch of sand. The preoccupied patron peeked at a comical clown hopping over the soft hot surface like a Mbenga fire walker and chuckled. Hold all calls meant instruments. The pungent smell of sterilized scrubbed surgical hand pieces, not the sweet smell of success, yet. The expensive Maquet 20 heart lung machine and a plethora of monitors were poised to assist in the best medical service money could buy. The buck stopped here, Taylor had often said. No American would be left behind or without. Now at the receiving end of the sermon he preached so often, so many theoretical scientific principles would once again come into play. The president was hurriedly prepped for the lengthy procedure.

Teams of specialists arrived, some merely to witness the awe inspiring procedure, still in shock. Spellbound by the secretive operation, rarely mentioned in the mainstream of respected medical journals, a whole other world waited for them to witness and explore. They found the hospital garb garish to say the least, not the usual lackluster pink or powder blue surgical scrub colors. The emblems emblazoned on the stunning attire with reflective silver streaks and 'racing stripes' suited the team well. A group of OR staff inscribed inside a small nothing it appeared in his line of work as he reluctantly answered the house phone. They'd track him down to the ends of the earth if need be he'd learned long ago.

"Uh huh, I see" he stated still fixated on the provocative postcard perfect posterior. "I arrived less than an hour ago, and you want me to what?" he pried the phone from his ear to prevent the shock wave from penetrating it. It sent his head spinning and out of the tranquil trance he tried to embed himself into.

"Haul your ass back here, ASAP!" snapped the voice on the other end of the line. "This is a state of national emergency."

"Yes, sir. The things I do for this organization.." and country he concurred as he caught one last glimpse of the compelling curvaceous form, if only a fleeting concept. He took a long hard swig from the tall cocktail glass, then set the cucumber slice next to it as if setting a wreath on a fallen soldier's grave. The mild mannered tourist, led anything but a mild or unimaginative existence. His manners left a lot to be desired. He'd learned to control his outbursts after the fateful scientific experiment that nearly 'atomized' his molecules. Yet the discovery of his 'metagenes', a mutation, a side effect still under intense military investigation and scrutiny, led to the unexplained superpower he was likely destined to acquire. He set the drink down. A waitress wiggled her hips enticingly snatched the empty glass and large tip from the table.

"Thanks" she said and admired his toned muscular torso as he pulled a polo shirt over it. She saw the strange logo for but a second, a splitting image of the one encountered ubiquitously in the Bethesda experimental surgical facility then left. His vacation plans utterly ruined once again. He needed a vacation from the vacations he'd had thus far. In his hotel room he hurriedly packed his US passport, Dr 'Sam' Palmer, a CMDF agent, and unassuming superhero hiding his identity well.

"Can't leave without this" he stated then reached for his belt, a brilliant stone embedded in the buckle. Neither like the bat utility belt, nor a wrestlers prize possession, but equally precious, priceless in fact. A rare element found only on a distant white star. The exact reason and time of it's discovery, still clear in his over active mind. He wound the belt through the loose holes around his long legged polo jeans. He made one last clean sweep of the room then caught a cab. Enroute Sam studied the large impediments still resting as they had since the 'stone age' at the side of the dirt road. The giant calcite stone wheels weighing several tons, were actually part of the Micronesian country's currency. The Rai or stone money. Such a ludicrously large immovable object, the larger the girth or circumference, the greater its monetary value. The largest came in at 628 stone, or 4 tons, 8800 lbs. Used as a form of barter, negotiating for a bride, an inheritance, or ransom, the currency had been in use almost as long, 500-600 years. The culture hadn't reinvented the wheel, only what it represented. Unlike Sam's experiments, which had fundamentally altered how we saw ourselves in this vast universe. Significantly smaller than presently perceived. He cast one last glance at the stone with the hole in the middle. He'd found it easier to pass through the eye of a needle while working then trying to crawl through the large circular stone coin during his leisure time. He reached YAP International departure lounge to

catch a Continental connector flight for the mainland. His flight arrived promptly, then bid adieu to paradise. One last look as the small baggage handler loaded his luggage. Marked 'Handle with Care', scientific samples from Guam University. The bulbous package was soon swallowed inside the belly of the beast bound for America.

Inside the elusive facility countless stories below DC, a submersible sat inside a large circular array of concentric lines radiating from the center of the circle, like a sundial or the brilliant rays of sun light. The odd nautical behemoth, with a bubble on top, a portal of some kind, sat quietly inside the space age carwash all spic and span. She'd received a wash, scrub down, rinse and final polish to a lustrous Turtle wax shine. The tired overtaxed technicians were performing a final walk about, assessing their pride and joy like an auto show aficionado. Awaiting her crew, the cleverly crafted concept, neither sub, nor boat, nor space vehicle, sat on display in the geometric grid of tiny hexagonal squares like a coveted revered queen bee. The technicians checked the delicate apparatus being loaded aboard the vehicle prior to departure.

"I knew his health wouldn't hold up. This IS our last hope, and it's a long shot" he stated apprehensively. Not a gambling man by any means, he'd rather not place a bet at the odds of even a remotely successful venture, if Jacques Cousteau were to pilot the craft himself.

The other technician studying the intake ports and polished brass hood ornaments took a different approach and attitude.

"TMR'll do the trick" he opted. "The president'll pull through. He's one tough nut to crack." They would soon find out literally what president Taylor was truly made of. The stuff of legends or lingering pockets of LDL lipoproteins and cholesterol. When both bypass surgery and angioplasty failed, Trans Myocardial Laser revitalization truly was the last resort. The technicians crawled through the cramped spaces aboard the sub. Packed with an odd assortment of carry on paraphernalia, they carefully placed the deceptively heavy 'beach ball' in a restraint.

"They'll get a 'kick' out of this!" chuckled the wiz kid. The recently developed soccer ball sized stem cell delivery system, was in actuality a giant C60 Bucky ball, or Buckminsterfullerene. A carbon based nanotubular network to carry the precious stash of cloned cardiac stem cells from the lab straight to the patient's heart. Marked 'Handle with Care' the curious sporty accessories served to while away the time in any foreign port or capital void of other pricier playthings and venues. In this case, the procurement process, years of painstaking work perfecting the stem cell line now missing only one component. A host heart, a specific site tailor made for this one of a kind spherical contraption. The contents enclosed in its elaborate skeletal framework much like the heart suspended in its rib cage radiating around it a protective practically impervious enclosure. They fastened the 'soccer ball' inside the tethered buffered receptacles like a kangaroo's pouch.

"As long as they remember which end is up" laughed the lead tech facetiously. He was correct of course, the deceptively round sphere, had only one opening, not the ideal poolside beach party receptacle to carry a cool can of refreshing Bud. Amazingly light, their foremost concern ever present. Inspite of the best contingency and simulated surgical practices, 'the best laid plans of mice and men gang aft agley' –Robert Burns. And if they indeed reach the target, the light as air beach balls, may get lost in the strong current ever present circulating through the patient's body. Their goal was to bring it to a snail's pace, a trickle in an as yet unproven, highly contentious procedure then bring the nuclear powered craft as close to the site of the damaged heart tissue as possible. Then a long roe to hoe as if planting a furrow for the following season. A good harvest and crop of meticulously nurtured cardiac stem cell 'seeds', to sprout and grow new vital vibrant cardiac muscle tissue that had been destroyed during the MI. The site of the scar tissue would stick out like a sore thumb, discolored, destroyed, depressed. It made the mission no less simpler. They still had millions of miles to go, a leap of faith, light years from the stone age flints, tools and natural salves used to cleanse and fix wounds back then.

2: Trick or Treat?

Annie Weinbauer: What have you done to your stereo?
Eddie Weinbauer: I wanted a new one.
(holding a bat over ruined stereo system)

- Trick or Treat, 1952
Disney cartoon

A dark limousine pulled up to a two story home in the trendy sleepy upscale suburbs of Chevy Chase and Friendship Heights in Washington, D.C. The night was always darkest just before the dawn, the street lights were still flickering. Two men departed from the black vehicle and swiftly positioned themselves outside the front door of the humble abode of one disgusted, disoriented dentist as he reached for the light switch. The door bell was rung relentlessly as he reached for the alarm clock to make the unbearable noise beating down on his eardrums stop. He noticed the time: 4 AM …the end of the world for all he cared. He wanted to roll over, but had to see who it was. Hopefully not the neighborhood brats again.

"Who the devil can that be?"

"You say something hon?" asked the alluring creature next to him as she rolled over slowly and provocatively. He prodded himself up just out of her reach then dashed out the door, down the stairs and peeked out the keyhole. The menacing grimaces in the pale moon light made him flinch. Hit men? Who could come knocking at this ungodly hour? The woman stretched her arm across the silky sheets, placed her palm flat on the smooth surface then waved it back and forth but failed to find the warm blooded all American male.

Reluctantly the riled recluse answered the door.

"Dr Gum?" asked the dark figure as he flashed some sort of ID card in front of the flustered fool's face. He couldn't focus. FBI, Local DC Metro police? The characters looked much more sinister. Mafia? Come to collect on an outstanding bill? He'd paid most of them on time.

"Yes?" he replied perplexed.

"Come with us" urged the dark figure. "It's a state of national emergency" he urged as they grabbed him under each arm about to drag him off. The woman covered the sheer wisp of a nightie with a terry cloth bath robe then crept to the staircase and stood there, startled, speechless.

"Can't it wait? Isn't this a job for the president?" he asked struggling to free himself. "Can I get dressed?" They couldn't wait and hauled him away.

"You'll be suited up when you get there" was all they said. The woman watched in horror. An odd way to show a token of appreciation, a promotion? A shopping spree? New designer duds he debated. He had put in many long hours lately at the office, seemingly 24/7.But it was still so early. Any stylish clothier opened their doors fashionably late, especially on weekends. What on earth could be so urgent?

"Do I have a choice?" he said latching onto a knob on the porch handrail on the way out.

"No!" they responded coldly, deliberately. They hustled him into the long black limousine like a rock star either enroute to his next concert or fleeing from the fans and mass exodus following a performance. The woman wondered where they were taking him and who he really was.

**

A world away a passenger jet soared into the outstretched arms of sunlight. The first rays reached over the horizon and frisked the fuselage. A warm welcome indeed. Midway down the rows, a medium build man, in his early thirties placed the dark rimmed sunglasses on his nose. The special lenses, part photogrey and a composite of rare earth and unknown elements filtered the dazzling flare like radiance of the sun as he lowered the tray in the seat in front of him. Sam placed the briefs in the confining small space, then flipped the folders carefully apart. 'Pyms's Particles', sub-atomic particle discovered, developed to induce size altering properties, then communicate with similar sized organisms. Blood born nanobots, to build parts, transform material endlessly inside the circulatory system. Miniaturization memos, mystifying manuscripts of international origin, countless countries and renown scientists. Who was the privileged passenger, an author, an agent, a spy? Had he stolen these documents? to trade them on the black market? To the highest bidder? He wondered if anyone else had seen these latest reports. The other side perhaps? As he perused several more highly coveted original copies. Elevated to almost a sacred status, the studies elaborated on the 'Buckminsterfullerenes', C60 balls. The file that followed was marked 'confidential top secret'. Had he saved the best for last? Or simply came up that way as he'd shuffled the deck hurriedly as he left the hotel. Stem cell implantation procedure for MI- myocardial infarctions, and other debilitating 'heart ailments'. The experimental procedure, the 'Stemwinder technique' . He scanned the laser script. The author a Dr Gum. Sam hadn't heard of him. No matter. The size and duration of the mission always varied.

"Can I get you anything, Dr Palmer?" asked the perky stewardess on a first name basis. She'd noticed a name tag or report as she repeatedly strutted her stuff down the narrow aisle. Her curiosity piqued. He wasn't the typical tourist or business traveler on a layover in the Micronesian playground she figured .

"No matter how many times I try to 'get lost' in Micronesia, they always manage to find me."
The shapely stew's demeanor swiftly changed. She thought family. Wife and children waiting back home. Though she'd been tempted before, she didn't want to rock the boat or rob the cradle.

"Your vacation plans cut short?" she probed cautiously.

"You might say...." Then drifted off in deep thought. "I'll have a Pimm's number 1. No make that a Maximum Voltage, hold the cucumber."
The suggestive reply sent her head spinning. Perhaps he was still an eligible bachelor. She rushed to the galley to prepare his cocktail personally. 50 ml Pimms No. 1, 25 ml Zubrowka vodka, an 25 ml Cointreau mint. The cucumber

rolled around the counter as she hurriedly returned with his drink, then waited as he fumbled with his briefs.

In the baggage compartment of the aircraft the item marked U of Guam, sat there silently foremost on the mind of the mysterious man.

**

The limousine maneuvered along the empty streets of the affluent upscale suburb bordering Maryland and DC. Dr Gum fought his urge to nod off on the smooth rolling ride that slowly lulled him to sleep.

"Where are you taking me?" he asked trying to strike up a conversation and common ground for the 'free ride', likely a heavy price to pay for the red eye excursion somewhere down the line.

"Ever heard of the CMDF?"

He thought long and hard for a few seconds.

"Comedic Mediation During Financial Fiascos?"

He looked at the zombie like blank stares opposite him in the sumptuous leather sofa then rephrased his reply. "Citizens Monitoring Deviant

unlike anything he'd ever seen in a museum, gallery or on TV before. Or had he? A golf cart came into his peripheral vision. Definitely not driven by Bob Hope or George Burns! The scientists and highly decorated military men, generals he guessed, invited him to hop on and tag along. Fearing he'd soon face Boris and Igor and/or the firing squad he complied and got on board the back seat of the tram. The golf cart hurried off down the tubular well lit metallic hallway. Not the early morning up before the crack of dawn round of golf he'd envisioned. The odd artificial light beginning to bother his blood shot eyes. A mini golf course? for select clientele? Must be. The cart came to an abrupt stop before a giant road block; a solid steel door to Ft Knox as far all he was concerned. The aging golfers, top ranking government officials by the look of ID cards and personal scans that revealed their most intimate credentials. The giant hermetically sealed door, nuclear bomb proof, he figured, rose. An entrance to a Norad like facility. Why had he been spared, not his girlfriend?

Inside the OR the president was prepped for the

delicate lengthy operation. Several specialists hurriedly assembled in the spur of the moment were escorted to the odd, ornate aerodynamic craft presumably for a test drive. The bubble on top, the large panoramic portal at the beak or front of the craft gave the invited guests the impression of a space craft or submersible. A high tech toy, nevertheless. A Christmas suggestion for a Saudi king perhaps or wealthy oil baron. But why him? wondered Dr Gum; definitely out of his price range. Several techs scoured the pointy 'grill' for bugs in the pseudo pre flight check and walkabout. Several marker or signal lights began to blink like a bloody UFO thought one of the startled senior scientists ogling the garish jalopy.

"All guidance systems go" informed the tech in a final show of confidence in the concept.

"Nuclear fuel topped up. She's good to go. 5 million miles to the gallon" he laughed. He just couldn't resist. A bubbly bodacious blond zipped up in a tight neoprene wet suit near the bow. She bent over to adjust her GPS ankle bracelet but found the controls confusing. The tech assisted in tuning into the correct frequency and 'station'.

The LED switch was working, yet,

"All dressed up and no place to go" he jested. She hadn't a clue where she was off to.

"Pam Cakes reporting for duty" she gushed with enthusiasm and exuberance, exuding a seductive sexual allure. The techs helped zip her up. It had taken some time to find a suit that fit.

"The navy never looked better" said the beet red tech not knowing where to place his hands to create some resistance and pull the stuck zipper up. Pam unzipped herself, still strategically concealing her ample cleavage then renegotiated the stressful suit up. Mission accomplished she approached the 'soccer balls' as if about to pump up and lead a group of nerdy high tech players to victory in a final match at Wemblay some day.

"Get a load of them balls" stated the technician, as Pam grabbed them and placed them against her curvaceous hips. The flustered techs were more concerned with following the bouncing balls then the task at hand. They nearly compromised the mission. The balls stuffed with anti cancer meds and cardiac stem cells,

"Uh, careful miss; don't want to blow 'em up too much!" he said intending no double entendre.

Pam carefully brought the bucky balls aboard and placed them in their pouches to await final placement like a pair of implants. Dr Gum was ushered into a changing area aboard, the locker room, along with a few renown team members.

Dr Mancini, the highly revered heart specialist and a pioneer of cardiac stem cell therapy. He'd performed the world's first organ transplant grown from the patient's own stem cells. One of the top cardio thoracic surgeons, was examining the patients charts. Like an ancient mariner perusing his nautical maps to lead them to a buried treasure on a distant shore. An eye patch suited him thought Dr Gum, the peculiar pirate type preoccupied with the navigational and surgical know how, planning the delicate operation from the inside. Pam, his pretty medical magician's assistant or wench? Which ever. It may take more than dumb blind luck to find the bull's eye he figured beginning to put the pieces of the puzzle together. The maps, medical charts, hurriedly created from MRI, CAT and CT scans and x-rays of the president's prostrate body. The 'road map' to guide, like the hitchhiker's guide to the galaxy for all he knew, to lead them to the damaged heart muscle.

"Ah, Dr Mancini, glad to have you aboard" acknowledged the studious staffer. The land lubber that he was, was eager to get an early head start, allowing him plenty of time to inspect the scar tissue.

"Guess I'll get my feet wet after all" as he ran his hands along the snug neoprene membrane. The novel approach to surgery completely foreign to him. He was along for the ride. Here for a good time, not a long time. They had their work cut out for them. Get in and out within the hour. He'd saved many a soul. The 'golden hour' in decisive trauma cases demanded the utmost in swift and precise motor hand skills. Heart transplants, angioplasties, shunts, stents, unclogging arterial plaque procedures he'd done thousands of, demanded no less attention to detail. He zoomed in on exploded diagrams of the patient's damaged arterial vessels and heart walls. It looked like a swampy murky blue bayou around Baton Rouge.

"This is commander Sparks. He'll be your pilot.

He was a former nuclear sub captain." No one was complaining yet. Eager to go where no man had gone before. Unfolding like a lucid dream, Dr Gum didn't know whether to pinch himself or roll over and go back to sleep. The crew were slowly introduced to one another to familiarize themselves with their fellow 'aquanauts'. Their lives would depend on each other's trust. The extent of their exploratory surgery anyone's guess at this juncture. They hadn't quite fathomed the far fetched concept and what little briefing they were given. Mostly grasping at straws and subtle clues along the way. Captain Sparks grabbed a few nautical charts like a crusty sea dog, then unfurled them onto the well lit counter, a bright exam light built into it from underneath.

"Doctor" stated Roger Sparks. With little more medical knowledge than bandaging a few radiation burns and scrapes aboard an LA class nuclear sub. He had to learn the lingo, and lead them through the murky uncharted territory in a flash so the skilled surgeon could get down to the dirty work. The president, the American people, the fate of the free world now rested squarely in the hands of the few sleepy chosen candidates. They did not know it yet though.

"Commander…" replied Dr Mancini extending his slender digits. They exchanged a firm hand shake.

"My assistant, Pam Cakes." The name, the comical relief Dr Gum referred to earlier, neither took the matter lightly, completely in stride.

"Looks like we're in good hands" she chuckled as she sized up the navigator and know it all smooth medical operator. She extended a hand and placed it on top of theirs, as if to say 'one for all and all for one'..then grabbed one of the x-rays. Repulsed by the angiograms, appalled at the clogged arteries.

"Good God, get a load of that plaque!"

"I'll admit…" Dr Mancini paused, then snatched the x-ray from her hand as if to steal her thunder. "He did enjoy those late night snacks."

Roger began with a philosophical statement, as if to set the tone for the entire eye opening journey. He eyed the unimaginably large bucky balls. How on earth the president would conceivably swallow his own words, 'the buck stops here' was still too difficult for the simple former merchant mariner to fathom.

"A man may esteem himself happy, when that which is his food is also his medicine." – Henry David Thoreau.

Inside the sophisticated nerve center, like a fully equipped OR, the spectators gathered in the gallery high above the operating theater. The naval personnel assembled at their computer stations like a team of NASA scientists anxiously awaiting the countdown, now moments prior to launch.

"T minus 5 minutes and counting" concurred the anxious analysts, calibrating the atomic clock above the theater. The surgical staff, scrub nurses and med students prepared for the lengthy operation. The implant itself the shortest albeit most prognostic indicator of the entire mission. A lengthy follow up contingency plan was in place in the event anything should God forbid go wrong, or the site of the scar tissue prove beyond repair. An escape route still in question. Where and how to extract the crew should they be stranded or forced to bail somewhere in the blood stream. A million questions brewed in the brilliant minds who'd used the quantum leap in technology only a handful of times prior to this. The most important perplexing problem to plague the staff, how to stop the heart, put the patient on bypass, the blood continuously perfused throughout his brain to prevent a permanent vegetative state. Not the vegetables the physicians had prescribed and harped on prior to the attack. To prevent a catastrophic implosion of the nuclear sub, Proteus, not only from the deafening thunderous roar of a beating heart, some 100,000 times in a day, 35 million in a year and about 2.5 billion in a lifetime. No more force than squeezing a tennis ball to force blood into the bloodstream, yet even one beat encountered during the delicate op could crush the sub like a Budlight can and squash the crew like bugs on a speeding bullet's windshield. No bigger than a few nanometers, the tiny nanobotic nautical medical mavens would have less than 30 minutes to complete the mission once inside the heart. Dr Gum began to slowly realize this was neither a trick in terms of slick doctored photography. He felt the cold smooth steel and hoisted his sorry ass up from the small seat in the change area. He crawled up into the 'bubble', curious. As he studied the gauges, he recognized the 'depth' meter rather than an altimeter. Must be a mistake. Several buoyancy gauges. Ballast? A submersible craft? To do the two step at the bottom of the Potomac? He climbed down the ladder than across the panoramic console to ceiling skylight. He took his place, alongside the other stupefied crew members, in his sumptuous snug leather seat, like an Indy racer strapped into a Recarro racing chair. It was all happening so fast. No way to turn back the hands of the clock now. Mutiny the only other option? He reflected on the words of a former president confined to his seat, sitting on 7.5 million pounds of lift off force TNT. 'Ask not what your country can do for you, but what you can do for your country.' - John F. Kennedy. Like astronauts or voyagers off to explore strange new worlds, to boldly go where no man had gone before, they awaited whatever fate was to be bestowed upon them. Less than a three hour tour? All were definitely in for a special treat as the technicians sealed the outer hatches and hurried from the nuclear submarine and the interior of the strange sophisticated chamber. The radiating concentric rings, lying under the novel nautical craft, like a bizarre launch pad. A mere push of a button sighed the speechless staff with baited breath. They eyed the atomic clock. It was time. Like a macabre memento left over from a future time and space, the surreal aerodynamic craft that may have visited the earth millions of years ago, rested ready to reach for the stars.

The crew anxiously awaited the next in what would no doubt be a memorable send off as the staff waved to the brave men and women, and closed the hatch, about to embark on the journey of a lifetime.

3: Secrets

'Nanotechnology will let us build computers that are incredibly powerful. We'll have more power in the volume of a sugar cube than exists in the entire world today.'

- Dr Ralph Merkle, molecular nanotechnology expert

Inside the submarine, the mood was solemn, the seconds now counting down to final launch. Dr Gum broke the ice and unwritten code of silence.

"What's all the commotion?' Someone die?"

Not up to speed, nor in the loop yet. The CMDF preferred to ease the candidates gently into the 'driver's seat' so to speak. And indeed, a patient, not just any patient, was clinging onto the last thread of hope in the adjacent theater. None of the crew had seen or even knew his whereabouts, prepped and resting comfortably on bypass. Bathed in the delicious elixir now sustaining his very existence, supplying his brain, vital organs and entire body with recycled yet continually freshly created RBCs; extracting the stale, used, carbon dioxide laden effluent. And as a precaution and matter of national security they would never directly come in contact with the president other than from a fresh novel perspective, inside Morgan Taylor, the 50th president.

Pam reached out her hand to the dumbfounded dentist and stem cell pioneer.

"Pam Cakes" she said with a contagious smile.

"It's a little early for breakfast, but I do believe in starting the day right with a healthy hearty meal." Surprised to see the stewardess on board, yet not a washroom nor a galley for that matter. This woman might know. Suffice it to say, she served as the perfect copilot or flying companion. The only way to fly, and a stew or cocktail waitress to boot.

"I'll have a 'stack' of pancakes, side of eggs, sunny side up, and a couple slices of bacon, toast and jam, freshly squeezed OJ and a coffee with cream to go with that." Pam looked about as if to say, 'can I take anyone else's order' then chuckled.

"I'm Pam Cakes…"

"Yes, I can see that" he nodded, like mister Magoo or Leslie Nielsen, on a one track mind, blind to the obvious, the buffoon introduced himself.

"Dr Gum."

Dr Dumb she thought, enchanted by the scatter brain.

"I'll be assisting Dr Mancini and yourself in the insertion of the stem cells into position…" she said provocatively. He was shocked to discover Pam was the alluring missing link in the medical mission. He wondered if she meant artificial insemination and what was next? He seemed to be the odd man out, out of the loop, learning on the fly. He hoped he'd have time to catch up since she came across as a former studious coed from college.

There was a slight delay in the mission. The staff worked feverishly to synchronize their time pieces essential for the success of the mission. There was still no sign of Sam. He'd been kept out of the loop too long to be an effective 'Plan B' figured the flustered techs.

It gave Pam a few precious moments to explain some of the ground rules to the buffoon. Out standing in his field, but if he tried anything, the first to be shoved off overboard in a rubber dinghy somewhere down the lazy river of blood.

He unfastened his seat belt as if to go to the washroom. He hadn't noticed a sign or door as of yet. Dr Gum passed the series of charts affixed to the light table his curiosity curiously aroused.

"All roads, uh arteries lead to Rome" he mused out loud. Pondering his appointment, performance thus far, and chance for a second term in office. The patient or origin of the congested 'traffic' hadn't crossed his mind. Pam got up from her comfortable resting position. Her high heels were beginning to bother her. She wanted to wear her crocs, but thought the whole story a croc, and utter fabrication by the two polite fellows who picked her up in the stretch limo. Producers? Certainly a novel approach to casting? They hadn't disclosed any details until a few moments ago.

"Looks like the I 395 northbound on the George Washington and Henry Shirley Memorial."

Pam decided to check the laser once more prior to departure. See that they hadn't overlooked a small detail. A Radio Shack not something they'd find once enroute. She fiddled with the switches.

"Watch your balls" she snapped. Pam aimed the scope at the center of the bucky ball, a large target by any stretch of the imagination. Not much larger than the head of a pin in the near future though. The flustered dentist jumped out of the way as a blast from the CO2 laser punched a hole in the prescription pad.

"Where's Sam?" wondered the technician.

"He's out of the country on vacation" said the commander sadly. They were truly on their own this time.

"He won't get here in time to assist in the operation?"

“Fraid not!”

Pam adjusted the tethers on the laser to insure it wouldn’t slip during unexpected turbulence swimming somewhere down that lazy river.

“A good man is hard to find” she stated mulling and reminiscing past loves lost. She’d made the right decision to leave her past behind and start over in high tech. Would it come back to haunt her? ‘The dance is a poem, each movement is a world.’ – Mata Hari, Dutch dancer, SS spy, one of the most famous espionage agents of all time.

**

In a dark deteriorating sector of the Severodvinsk naval yard, the 2nd largest ship yard in the world; once the pride of the Russian navy, now a derelict run down remnant of the former glory dating back to Imperial Russian rule. A bright flash, like a shooting star, or aurora borealis filled the night sky over the remote northern naval center. All the rules had been literally thrown out the window in an instant as a select sector of former Soviet KGB agents and government defectors watched and waited anxiously. The bright lights encompassing the small fleet of vessel, like a Hollywood premiere or enlightening christening of a new novel addition to the fleet continued to illuminate the waters directly below the vessels. From above the band of bright ‘flood lights’, neither a holographic projection, something you might see during a David Copperfield magic trick, slowly enveloped the flotilla, nor a helicopter search light scoped the docks for smugglers pilfering rapidly rusting parts, fetching a pretty penny on the Russian black market. Prized and horded in such high volumes, the officials figured they could retrofit or produce an entire battle cruiser from spare parts. The lights radiated unlike any search or floodlight, focused on an entire contingent of fast frigates and cruisers.

As if undergoing an intense scan by a massive Russian MI 24 or even significantly larger aircraft, or extensive x-ray scanner, neither portable nor compact. For a few split seconds the fleet was there.

The commander nodded his head, as if to signify a final fateful execution, or carriage of justice. A firing squad? The holographic beams focused on the fleet. In the ensuing seconds, there were none.

The entire battle fleet had disappeared. A nuclear blast? Inconceivable, the country had clamped down on illicit plots to penetrate the secure limited nuclear stash that remained. A special effect? A Russian or foreign film crew hard at it in the great white north of Russia?

A scientist in a white coat picked up what resembled a miniature toy replica of a Russian cruiser very carefully. In turn each of the convoy was transferred to a square 'aquarium', half full of a liquid, either salt water or some form of slick preservative. He slid a cover slide over the top and gently placed it onto the tines of a fork lift. The vehicle slowly maneuvered the cube toward was could only be described as a helicopter pad. Yet in lieu of the usual, the letters 'GRU' appeared around a series of concentric rings like a bull's eye. The same military intelligence logo or decal GRU was found ubiquitously on the soldier's shoulder padded suits, the vans, and most of the military paraphernalia.

The scientists hurriedly cleared the landing pad. The bright lights beamed down onto the 'cube'. It rapidly began to shrink to the size of a 'sugar cube'. Then darkness descended upon the deceptive decrepit remote district of the naval yard. Several men bearing the emblem GRU, actually the 4th department, the headquarters also known as 'The Aquarium', the top secret central agency of the Russian military intelligence agency. It employed hundreds of thousands, many former KGB agents, assassins and so forth.

The sugar cube, now miniaturized and hermetically sealed was gently hoisted from the landing pad and gently dropped into a bottle of the best Russian vodka, then capped and resealed. The cube remained relatively stable inside the crystal clear contents of the liquid. As if weighted like a magic 8 ball. The scientists were hustled inside an MI8 helicopter then whisked off to a 'restricted zone' escorted by heavily armed MIGs and MI 8 helicopters. The team arrived on the outskirts of the capitol. In a secure suburb, a cluster of bland buildings served as the GRU headquarters. The runway was partially obscured, obstructed by a perimeter defense system to protect top secret experimental military aircraft and helicopters.

"Take them to 'the Aquarium.'

"Da."

The men bearing a priceless gift were hurried into the heavily defended facility. They passed several check stops and security clearance points like an airport custom's border station, never once asked about the bottle of 'booze'. Satisfied they were escorted into the inner hive. Ironically in the 'GRU' complex lay an exact replica of the under ground CMDF facility in Bethesda, DC. Once again proving the counter intelligence KGB predators had and continually did pilfer, then reverse engineer many American military secrets after the cold war.

"Prepare our little 'token of appreciation' for the Americans. The bottle was placed once again onto a small elevated podium which rose from the intricate tiled floor bearing a series of concentric rings. As the floor lit up like a 80's disco dance floor, the bottle reduced to the size of a small mini bar selection found in any hotel room in a country consuming the beverage anywhere in the 'free' world. The fleet now in suspended animation, hermetically sealed in its own little universe, presumably in some sort of weighted vacuum, like a system of gimbels to prevent a catastrophic communist capsizing. The woman presented the bottle as a gesture of gratitude to the top GRU agent assigned to the delicate operation. He took the highly coveted bottle and placed it inside his briefcase, as part of his only declared carry on items then departed to carry out his highly orchestrated covert op. He stopped briefly on the tarmac and looked around and to smell what was only the toxic aviation fuel fumes then boarded the aircraft.

"This precision operation is going to drive me to drink comrade" came a reply from a startled soldier, roughly translated from the Russian.

"Da", acknowledged his stunned subordinate.

**

The CMDF was a beehive of activity like Mission Control in Houston prior to launch. The generals paced back and forth nervously as the crew secured themselves in their seats. Roger Sparks climbed up under the small dome and waved to the technicians who gave the thumbs up outside. They'd waited what seemed like an eternity to test their new toys and the latest methods to embed the miniaturized stem cells, that had been amplified millions of times over to create the 'bucky' ball sized desired dose. Sparks peered about his omnidirectional bubble then closed his eyes and said a little prayer.

The generals gave the green light and go ahead. The atomic clock began to count down each nano second as the bright lights began to bombard the nuclear submarine.

Simultaneously in the adjacent operating theater, the surgeons prepared to let the president's heart take a breather. With the aid of a Da Vinci surgical robot, they placed a few tiny 'keyhole' incisions to prep the heart to allow the deoxygenated blood from the SVC and IVC to be carried out to the Maquet HL 20 heart lung machine and do all the dirty work for president Taylor. The blood thinner heparin was added to the HR 20, then oxygenated, cooled. It slowly advanced into the ascending arm of the aorta. A slow, steady flow at about 4-5 l/min., sufficient to perfuse vital brain and organ tissue. Yet a horrific torrent to any adversary or antibody flowing inside the circulatory system.

"'Be still my beating heart'" stated the surgeon, ready to rock and roll. The object of his affection and obsession throughout his medical residency. He could only imagine what it'd be like from the driver's seat inside the sub, more like a raging river, an Indy or Nascar raceway, bound to be a few bumps and bruises along the way. A fatal 'crush' injury foremost on his mind should the president's heart resume its usual duty, likely always at an accelerated pace. He preferred to approach the problem from his highly trained hands and eye's and mind's perspective as he rehearsed the delicate contingency plans a few times pending the out come of the mission. He'd know in less than an hour if he'd have to take evasion action and pursue a more aggressive approach and/or have to extract the crew by a radical emergency measure. Either course of action potentially fatal to the president.

The OR nurse wiped the sweat from his brow. The surgeon, center stage, was eager to get on with it, his learned colleague, the unassuming anxious anaesthetist quietly blended into the backdrop. He'd settled into a peaceful composed posture after administering the initial meds. Only a few seconds of sheer terror at the end bringing the patient back, marked by an hour of R & R if everything went according to plan. He scanned the ECG, EKG, O2 pulse oximeter, all within normal range for a heavily sedated patient, about to undergo the life threatening novel bypass stem cell therapy. The first lady and White House staff was continuously instantly informed of the state of the president.

The joint chiefs of staff were pacing nervously in front of a live feed from the operating room at the CMDF center.

"We haven't lost a president on my watch." The veteran armed forces commander felt totally powerless in the current state of affairs. So far removed from the front lines of battle, and beyond even his brilliant military mind. He could only imagine what natural let alone man made adversaries and obstructions the crew may encounter along the way to their objective, literally to the heart of the matter. He checked his Omega watch and noted the time.

"He's certainly not going down without a fight" fumed the first lady defiantly, as if facing a formidable foe herself from her husband's vantage point. "The stress was too much. It finally got to him." The general held her tightly, reassuring her, "You've stuck by his side through thick and thin, he's a fighter, he'll pull through this."

"Thank you for your vote of confidence" she stated cracking a weak smile.

A barrage of pesky reporters filled the press room hanging on any and all updates and snippets of information the press secretary may dish out.

The operation had entered a delicate, dicey phase. The perfusionists pushed the heparin through the heart lung machine to prevent clotting. The blood had been chilled to 28-32 degrees C (82.4 - 82.9 F), to slow the metabolic consumption rate, still a balmy bordering on tropical jacuzzi temp for the four skin divers. The blood traced an intricate 'mouse trap' route through the labyrinth of lines and series of 5 pumps to and fro from the patient. The reservoir, a trap, to extract the crew in case of an emergency extraction, the only logical escape route reasoned the perfusionist and surgical staff prior to departure. Through the oxygenator, heated, then squeezed through a series of rollers to push it into the patient. Five rollers insured the blood found its way back to the machine to continue the mundane repetitive life support route.

"Begin miniaturization, take her down to sub level 1" commanded the admiral.

"Miniaturization sub level 1" repeated the programmer like a parrot.

The bright lights bombarded the sleek sub. It began to shrink slowly at a steady rate. The rings like those of a tall evergreen continued to encircle the craft as it shrunk. The bewildered staff, many witnessing the event for the first time, counted the circles. Their heart's racing, likely the number of years they'd lose after the harrowing high tech procedure were over.

Inside the Proteus, the crew felt no change to their systems already racing in adrenaline over drive. They were stunned by the rapid reduction of their measurements. The biggest losers? In the land of the giants. The light show ceased temporarily.

"Makes you feel rather small and insignificant"

sighed Pam as she peered out of the vessel. "But big enough for my bubble bath" she imagined equating the incredible shrinking machine to a tiny submersible electric toy mischievously.

The crew continued to watch in amazement as everything 'grew' to gigantic proportions outside the panoramic port.

"Raise platform."

"Raise platform" reiterated the veteran staffer. A small hexagonal podium or pedestal rose from the center of the circular bull's eye. It looked like a trophy showcase thought the retired admiral from the situation room. A token of appreciation for years of service to the navy. It brought a tear to his eye as he reminisced about his lengthy career from cadet rising to the rank of rear admiral. A slight jolt rocked the vessel as two tiny tine of a forklift type device elevated the sub onto itself. They were now suspended in mid air high above the circular theater as the podium retracted down into the floor. Center stage, like a flying trapeze act, any move death defying potentially catastrophic.

"Free as a bird" marveled Roger as he peered over to the forklift driver, paying meticulous attention to the transfer.

"I'm still in awe" mentioned Dr Mancini still unable to comprehend the transformation. "about the 'transition' to inner space. a mini nuclear sub… and I'll soon be no bigger than one of the nanobots that I use in my microvascular surgeries…" he stated shaking his head.

"No bigger than a menacing microbe" noted Roger as he perused the controls.

"What about antibodies and macrophages?" wondered Dr Mancini, worried about the size of any formidable foes.

"I wouldn't worry about 'them'," stated Sparks. "We've got an hour."

"Then what?" replied the medical specialist.

"Then I'd worry" stated Sparks facetiously, chuckling nervously. Hopefully they'd finish the task and fled well within the golden hour.

"We'll grow logarithmically" added Pam precociously.

"This is where I get off" stated Dr Gum still unable to fathom the concept, unaware of the occupational hazards. No one had filled him in on the finer details. He unlatched his shoulder harness about to bolt for the escape hatch.

Pam reattached his harness tightly.

"It's OK, you can swim can't you?" She was certain the crew met minimum admission's requirements.

"Yes, but…"

"You'll be fine."

A giant glass vessel was slowly rolled into position center stage just below the sub. The giant cylindrical aquarium still more than a several meter high springboard from the sub. More like a cliff dive, or fatal crash from the lofty height.

"Time for your bath" quipped the technician facetiously as he gently lowered the sub onto the rim of the glass and removed the forklift tines.

"Splish splash" stated Pam, then giggled. The subtle jolt shocked them as the vessel rocked gently on the surface of the reservoir.

"Activating ballast tanks one and two" stated Sparks then flipped a few switches which let out the ballast. A green light came on the console followed by a surge of champagne bubbles or obnoxious flatulence underneath the belly of the beast depending upon the interpretation of each crew member. The Proteus slowly sank into the sunset, in the relatively dark theater prior to the brilliant blast of light during the opening act. The bubble dome quickly covered in the saline solution and continued to sink. The forklift left the circle, the podium slowly settled back into the floor, leaving a slight sick feeling in the pit of the stomachs of the landlubber's amongst them. A slight queasiness and vertigo accompanied the drop. Much milder than the drop of doom at a Disney world attraction, but no less dangerous.

"Begin miniaturization level 2."

"Level 2 miniaturization."

The bright lights bathed the room once again. A brilliant kaleidoscope of colors emanated outside the large portal, slightly mitigated. Pam preferred a set of Ray bans to shield her eyes from the radiant light but wasn't warned ahead of time to properly pack for the occasion. Certainly not the tropical getaway she'd hoped for.

4: Take the Plunge

> 'Agnes Darling, if such should be we never meet again, while firing my last shot, I will gently breathe the name of my wife – Agnes- and with wishes even for my enemies, I will make the plunge and try to swim to the other shore.'
>
> - Wild Bill Hickok, lawman, gunfighter, scout

The Proteus, and the glass vessel slowly shrunk to the size of a hypodermic cylinder. Dr Mancini had grasped the gravity of their miniaturization process and could only imagine the size of the plunger necessary to propel the tiny radioactive marker into the patient. Hopefully in a large muscle mass like the gluteus maximus. Not a pretty picture he thought, preferring to meet the president if ever granted the opportunity, face to face, tete a tete during a friendly fiesty state dinner or RSVP. Time permitting, nothing short of a jugular juxtaposed entry point to reach the heart, he'd calculated. The naval commanders of the CMDF preferred a safer entry point in the radial or ulna, the arteries feeding the forearms, the standard patient hospital infusion site practiced daily by the ER staff.

"Elevate platform."

"Elevate platform" came the echo like parroted reply. The miniscule dose of stem cells dwindled with each progressive phase. The sub no larger than the head of a pin now, the syringe ready to receive the brunt of the blow to proceed to the target. Another small retractable, movable arm rotated around a pivotal point to grab the radically reduced glass cylinder. A plastic rubber tipped plunger was slowly depressed into the end of the opening. It rested there snug in it's receptacle. They were about to enter the operative phase of the elective surgery. President Taylor's reelection chances equally hung in the balance of the brilliant surgical team about to come to terms with his mortality. They'd know within 57 minutes if he had survived the first round of the primary procedure. A second tense nail biter if the sub's stem cell intervention failed.

The syringe was delicately delivered into the adjacent op as if transferring a freshly harvested donor organ. The OR nurse prepared to gently puncture the swabbed landmark on the president's forearm. The video cameras zoomed in. The radial artery was missing, removed from a previous CABG, coronary artery bypass graft. It left only one alternative, the ulna, now the direct route straight to the heart, it reduced the margin of error significantly. The sub could not conceivably get lost? or could it? An ominous silence befell the operating theater. One could hear a pin drop. The consequences, a potential catastrophe if the submarine were to venture near the semicircular canals, like a tourist missing their turn off on a California turnpike.

The president was now well under, as the anaesthetists closely monitored him to maintain a still somnolescence. The sound of the rollers pushing the blood back into his body through the oxygenator, into the SVC, superior vena cava and IVC, inferior vena cava, in an endless loop set the stage. The perfusionist satisfied the blood heparin thinner was at the desired level, ushered the team in. The hydraulic instrument cart was gently wheeled into the OR.

"All set to sail?" asked the perfusionist enthusiastically. The robotic doc dispensed the desired angle and trajectory of the tiny nuclear projectile. The scrub nurse position the impact or entry site directly above the landmark, denoted by a small bull's eye.

Inside the Proteus, the crew sat on pins and needles anxiously awaiting their 'shot' at saving the president's life.

"The president truly is larger than life" chuckled Pam, "he's a lot bigger than I imagined from all the Fox reports" she ribbed as she peered out over the vast hairy vista akin to the rain forest from her eagle's eye vantage point.

"All systems go" signaled the knowledgeable team of naval and nuclear engineers. They scanned the cluttered consoles with baited breath.

"Let us proceed" said the commander confidently saying a little prayer softly. All eyes then bounced back to the large circular atomic clock and back to the OR.

"Bon Voyage!" bid the nurse to her tiny entourage then depressed the plunger.

The Proteus suddenly surged forward down a long smooth dark tunnel with blinding speed. The crew were pushed into their seats, pinned by the sudden unexpected g forces. Similar to a Cape Canaveral rocket launch, yet slightly smoother. The narrow channel or smooth contours of the hypodermic left little leeway as they raced toward the small angled aperture at the end of the tip, immersed somewhere inside the president's forearm. Pending a clean puncture wound, they'd soon find themselves sailing along the 'lazy river' of blood. Pam gripped the armrests amazed by the sudden surge, infinitely more shocking than the log ride drop of doom at Knott's Berry Farm, the only comparable reference point.

Sparks watched in wonder as the tiny world of turbulent eddies danced about over his head. He peered ahead to the distant darkening virtual horizon, a sliver at the end of the stainless steel tip where it pierced the president's venule muscular rings. He braced himself for impact unable to gauge what it may seem or feel like. This was all so fascinating and incredibly new to the crew, as they sat there, their faces torn between smiles and sheer terror.

"He'll be on heart lung bypass for 30-90 minutes" gauged the veteran cardiovascular trauma surgeon if all went well. "If we need to go in, we will" he stated. He'd cross that bridge if he had to. Their mission, to bridge the gap of dead scar tissue in the heart, and patch it with viable totipotent cardiac stem cells. Never been done before, sheer conjecture at this juncture.

"That will give them enough time to locate the clogged coronary artery near the previous infarct site, lase it, then implant the stem cells" reiterated the commander to insure they were all on the same page. He looked up at the clock. So little time, so much to do. A three hour tour compressed into a few fleeting seconds. Certainly not a pleasure cruise albeit all the sights and sounds never seen before by tourists or talented team of specialists ever before. He walked up to the map of the president's arm. The nuclear sub's stream of effluent, like a radioactive tracer, gave him their coordinates every step of the way. The tiny blip about to make 'landfall' in the lower arm of president Taylor. He looked up at the clock once again then up to the heavens… "God willing, swim like spawning salmon upstream and out the ascending aorta back down to the ulnar arteries to the palmar digital to the tip of the finger if I understand you correctly, Dr Mancini."

The Proteus shot through the tip of the hypodermic. The long angular slit sat midstream in a relatively weak cross current. Marked by countless little circular 'lifesavers' as Pam so comically described them. The sub swerved to avert direct impact with the opposite wall of the blood vessel. Dr Mancini and the rest of the crew were startled by the lack of the familiar 'lub dub', and steady back beat of the blood. Merely a slow meandering river, the perfusionist maintained at 4-5 l/min.

Sparks set a course 'upstream', full speed ahead. Dr Mancini caught in a moment of shock and awe as he peered out of the front of the sub. The tiny blue bubbles of deoxygenated blood, danced and swirled about the sub, a relatively large impediment to their unrestricted playful antics.

"You got it General. As easy as performing a finger prick! All you have to do is remove us in a drop of 'tagged' blood, then deposit us onto a microscope slide." The surgeon listened to what he said. The gravity of the concept still hadn't sunk in. No squeamishness was detected in his confident brash and bold demeanor that denied any margin for error. The smooth operator had lost only a few patients, beyond repair. He placed his chances as 'favorable', yet much of the mission was still well out of his hands. Dr Mancini had to rely on the experienced nuclear sub commander just to get him to the operating site.

"Like a radioactive labeled marker..assuming we're all aboard the nuclear sub" surmised the mystified dentist as he peered at an image of the remote OR. Their presence merely a speck of dust, that had disappeared inside the arm of the virtual patient. The map, a highway marked by twisting turning, winding roads. A lone dashboard light, a beacon of hope on the informative highway, inched along up to the turnpike, a hairpin turn at the president's shoulder. They were still 'hundreds of miles' relatively speaking from the target. Pam ran her hand along her ankle bracelet, the only other ID, should they be forced to abandon ship and be separated in the current, or swept 'ashore' inside a layer of epithelial cells lining the wall of the blood vessels. Her transponder seemed to have malfunctioned. She smiled nervously as the men averted their attention from the map to study her curvaceous anatomy.

"Yes.." acknowledged the commander. He preferred not to dwell on the unthinkable, ditching or bailing before they even reached the target. Pam was getting cabin fever and restless already.

"Pitter patter, let's get at 'er" she urged impatiently pacing about nervously. She preferred they 'reach the beach' or some other exotic foreign shore that she'd always imagined she'd set foot on. Like a lab rat seeking a way out, she soon began to get on Spark's nerves. The commander was concerned that the craft was moving along at a snail's pace. Had they overestimated the craft's negotiation of the seemingly endless network of long veins? Had the CMDF miscalculated their elapsed time to the target? Their ETA still seemed like hours away. They had to get a move on. He couldn't jettison any flotsam or jetsom, especially not the laser to lighten the load and increase their chances of getting to the coronary site on time. He adjusted the angle of attack, and veered midstream. The decrease in peripheral venule wall resistance caused a noticeable surge in the speed of the sub. He breathed a sigh of relief and reasoned by tweaking their trajectory continually, they'd hopefully reach their objective on time. The sooner the better. Their means of escape no walk in the park by any stretch of the imagination.

Roger was spellbound by the sheer beauty of the bizarre blood borne objects, like globules of jelly fish, some transparent, a bluish tinge, tossed about in an erratic water ballet.

"Fascinating! Just as the body cannot exist without blood, so the soul needs the matchless and pure spirit strength of faith'," (-Gandhi) he sighed in wonder.

"There's a lot of blood, sweat and guts between dreams and success" stated Dr Gum pragmatically. An amateur sailor from his senior years, still found it difficult to fathom where they were and how they were going to implement the remedy.

"God gave man both a penis and a brain, unfortunately not enough blood supply to run both at the same time" (Robin Williams) chuckled Pam. She could only imagine how much blood supplied the rest of the president's body.

"De humana corporis fabrica, the fabric of life, the human body". Each in their own little world of wonder. Bringing with them their personal past and experiences. This unlike anything they could've ever imagined. The sense of sheer delight soon transitioned to one of urgency as the seconds ticked by.

"A stitch in time saves nine" said Pam then took a head count. … "uh four." In any event she recognized they were rapidly running out of time, and they hadn't even reached a number of check points. The checkered flag still far off on the distant horizon.

"We'll beeline for the basilic vein then enter the subclavian and on into the SVC" stated the man up in the bubble, like a bewildered boy scout at his first jamboree or pacman tournament. The lack of a pulse propelled the tiny projectile rapidly forward as he got the hang of the delicate navigational requirements. Rather than bouncing off the walls, the captain, continued to set a course through the imaginary slalom gates or buoys he set in his mind's eye. "….smooth sailing. It's a vast improvement since our maiden voyage" declared the dedicated pilot.

Dr Mancini scanned the meticulously detailed map. Like a bathyspheric or underwater topographical chart, the surface terrain painted a gloomy picture. The president's over indulgence in the finer things in life, likely countless late night snacks, had done seemingly irreversible damage. The irregular contours and rocky shoals, were the clogged arteries of arteriosclerotic plaque affixed to the walls of the cliffs or blood vessels like massive barnacles.

"Got himself in a bit of a sticky wicket" suggested Dr Gum equating the rough patches as plaque on an other wise smooth tooth surface. Ideal sites for bacteria and microorganisms to latch onto. The dirty work had been done. He'd literally dug himself a grave, down in the depths of Davy Jones locker.

"I'll say. Not as ship shape as we initially thought he was. Like you said, I haven't seen such a traffic jam since they opened Yankee Stadium" in a desperate attempt to inject some light hearted humor into the unfolding drama.

"I hear he likes to go to watch the Nationals play" said Pam, prompting some speculation and palliative measure, even a placebo perhaps if the situation warranted it mused Dr Mancini.

"They'll be takin' him out to the old ball game in a body bag if we don't repair that dead heart muscle!" stated Dr Mancini prognostically. "2 out" he discounted CABG and angioplasty. "2 strikes", including stroke and myocardial infarction. "bases loaded" referring to the occluded blood vessel blockage, “bottom of the ninth…” he looked at the dismal scenario and deliberated. “We’ve all he’s got. We’re his last best chance!”

The despondent heart specialist fidgeted nervously, helpless to intervene, powerless to procure a remedy from his present position as he loomed larger than life over the charts, mapping out his plan of attack amidst the cardiomyopathic mess. He was left with little margin for error. He only hoped he’d hit this one out of the ball park!

“ETA to the heart, 20 min” sounded Sparks.

By the CMDFs calculations, that left one half hour. Ten minutes to work and 10 minutes to escape. A carefully choreographed scheme of events that cut it close, too close for comfort figured the rest of the crew. Dr Mancini offered his optimistic opinion.

“That’ll give us plenty of time to poke around, lase the injured muscle and replace it with totipotent cells. Then the president can give us the bird for all I care…” he quipped, the tip of the middle finger blood the planned escape route. The others didn’t share the same sense of morbid medical humor.

In the CMDF mission control center, the staff watched the illuminated blip inch up the president's arm. In the OR, his vitals remained steady and stable, the Maquet heart lung machine purred softly, the rollers running along repetitively pushing the life saving liquid through president Taylor's heart.

"How are his vitals?" asked the commander from the eye in the sky overlooking the OR.

The staff scanned the series of monitors spewing out a steady stream of data much to the delight of the surgeon.

"Stable, within normal range. He's a fighter" he offered if only a placebo. "He'll feel a little light headed after the operation" he stated pending a successful closure to this chapter of his term in office. He didn't want to belabor them with needless details. Perfusion always permeated the pronounced folds of brain tissue less than optimally. By the same token, perfusion created pooling of blood in the heart due to the reduction in speed and efficacy of complete transfer of deoxygenated blood. A minor inconvenience, tolerable, and not necessarily life threatening.

The valves dispersed throughout the venous return system at intermittent intervals came up fast for the sub captain. The gaping gaps closed suddenly like a giant whale's gaping orifice. In lieu of baleen, the elastic muscle mass could trap the sub in its grip, potentially leaving them stranded, high and dry, pinned inside the small venule. Like a giant wine press, the walls constricted, causing a potentially fatal 'crush' injury for the crew of the Proteus. They poised and paused occasionally and looked up to the pilot under the plastic bubble. In good hands thus far as he followed his heart and navigational compass closer to the scene of the accident.

The White House was abuzz. The DoD, joint chiefs of staff, paced about the large table in the situation room. Instant live feed like a live communication's satellite intelligence link gave them the head's up.

"Just make sure, you keep us 'in the loop'," urged the first lady, eyeing the intricate sophisticated apparatus. She was briefed by the White House physicians about the workings of the heart lung machine. She knew her husband was literally at the mercy of the machines. Relying on the rollers of the pump to perfuse his blood vessels and organs as urgently as the press secretary provided up to date information of the various organizations and press reporters waiting with baited breath about his status. All in due course she conceded.

"Aye aye ma'am" replied the mission commander promptly. She expected to be informed immediately of any alterations to his health. She had to have a clear picture in her mind, in order to know what and how much to release so as not to upset and lay to rest any rumors a curious public had that spanned the globe.

A barrage of obnoxious reporters were suddenly disturbed by a rapidly developing situation. The president's predicament and current status on a slippery slope; had someone leaked his precarious position to the paparazzi wondered the staff. The breaking news story meant only one thing, 'trouble a brewin' .

"Turn it up a notch!" demanded the department of defense chief of staff.

5: Gruesome

> "A gruesome thought, then it grew some more."
>
> - Dr Gum, dentist, crew member of mission

All eyes turned to the breaking Fox broadcast on the large flat screen at the front of the situation room.

"A terrorist faction…with possible ties to Al Qaeda claims to have swiped a few of the Russian 'briefcase' nukes." He pushed the earphone into his left ear, trying to mute the mob gathered about him. The caption read somewhere inside Washington D.C. A clever ploy by the networks to distract the public from the president's precarious predicament? The White House had issued no press releases nor been brought up to speed on any recent rebellious uprisings. The first lady fiddled with the remote and raised the report audibly. "…as many are reported missing as are missiles pointed at Washington" he stated. To corroborate his claim he introduced a middle aged, man form the crowd. "With us is former GRU defector, Dmitry Lebedev…"

"The TSA checks all carry ons, the airports are practically airtight. Thank God" she fretted yet the sum of all her suspicions could not be sequestered.

"Mr Lebedev, can you tell us what was in that briefcase?" The noted nuclear counter terrorist, and former special delivery operative for the Russian military intelligence network knew all too well what was lost. Certainly what was at stake. He slowly gained his composure amongst the noisy crowd as if auditioning for a film, a spy thriller perhaps? He slowly peered intently into the camera. His fiery eyes like that of Rasputin instilled the fear of God into the viewers. He cut right to the chase.

"A small nuclear device…" he paused to gather his breath, noticeably upset. "The RA115's or RA115-01's, the submersible variant, weighing about 50-60 lbs." The words submersible struck a chord with the first lady. She sequestered the unimaginable.. brought aboard the submarine? Impossible. The crew and secure facility were checked meticulously, prescreened for clearance. "They remain active for years. With the explosive force of a W54," the American equivalent, "6kton of TNT". The bombs dropped on Hiroshima or Nagasaki were 16-21 kton. "..and a lighting trigger device, several KGB ad GRU agents brought them into the country to annihilate entire cities and to assassinate US officials and citizens."

A contingent of heavily armed rebels raided and stormed the secure Russian facility at the outskirts of Moscow. They rapidly overran the respectable military resistance. The carefully choreographed plan was pulled off without a hitch. An inside job?

The counter terrorists resistance receded. The officials were quickly herded to the chamber bearing the large bull's eye of concentric rings radiating from the center of the room. A far cry from the camel back raiders or stone age cave dwellers. The stunned staff, petrified, their fingers poised at various positions above their control consoles as if in suspended animation, choked,

"What do you want?" asked a feisty fellow of the Russian Academy of Sciences.

The infiltrators demanded they get up from their desks very slowly, nice and easy, insuring them no one would get hurt. They then herded the entire staff of specialists and scientists into the large vacuous space.

The rebel leader quickly opened all channels to communicate with his captive audience. He seemed to know his way around the control room like a late night disc jockey at a local Moscow radio station. The scientists huddled around on top of the cluster of concentric rings. They hadn't the foggiest how and who led the charge. The Kremlin would certainly soon get wind of the madmen's motives. They knew they couldn't escape. They hadn't considered the consequences of standing center stage. The three ring circus performance about to begin. Without further ado, he cut to the chase.

"Consider yourselves taking a permanent leave of absence from the 'inner space race'," he stated loud and clear. The rebel leader nodded. The gunmen hurriedly exited the room, locking it from the outside barring any chance of escape.

He then flipped a few switches as if to begin a live recording session at a studio. They shielded their eyes from the bright blast of light radiating around the room, above the bewildered scientists and directly below their feet. They'd soon sample a taste of their own experimental medicine. A bitter pill to swallow. And likely soon too large to taste. The stunned staff were soon reduced in more than rank as they disappeared from sight. A swift miscarriage of justice, far more efficient than the firing squad, figured the mad man at the helm. Firing meant full and complete erasure from the earth as he set the controls on an endless loop of miniaturization. The staff were literally 'atomized' ultimately to nothing more than black matter, the ether or glue holding the galaxies together. The rest of the terrorists could not fathom the concept. Out of sight was as good as out of mind.

"Round up the others!" demanded the demented rebel. The scientists in other sectors of the building were urged to 'take a break' and follow the fiends. Downsizing had taken on a whole new meaning in the renown Russian military center. Hordes of scientists were handed their resignation, without a fight, on a silver platter.

"A gruesome thought!" uttered the first lady.

"You can't be serious?" snapped the skeptical CNN reporter. "Russia's Atomic Energy Commission denies their very existence."

The Russian spy laughed into the camera.

"Not only are they very real, but our own miniaturization forces found a way to conceal, ie shrink, them for several hours to avoid detection." Why, you could be carrying one aboard in that microphone" he chuckled then erupted into a crazed cackle. The stunned Fox reporter looked at his mike. "Why at this very moment a GRU agent could be coming to the steps of the White House to present an ‘iron clad’ proposal for the president in person…” he played with the heart strings of the captive audience, now many hundreds of millions watching the emergency broadcast being briefed about the unbelievable. It sounded like some thing out of a science fiction film.

“Then it grew some more…” stated a stunned joint chief of staffer. Spellbound, speechless. Stunned by the fact the Russians had the same technology, and trumped them by taking it to the next level, extending the length of the mission. How they had gotten a hold of the coveted technology beyond him. The KGB and GRU must’ve done their homework he figured. Who had turned it over posed another pressing question. It seemed no one could be trusted any more! A million thoughts crossed his mind. How to secure the White House, the capitol region? The airports? How could they conceivably scan for such surreptitious insertions into the country? Inconceivable. A wake up call, it certainly kicked the international game of espionage up a whole notch or two. The Potomac two step, no longer for the privileged few in the CMDF. The technology fallen into enemy hands, gave the Russians a chance to tango in this tangled web of deceit and counterintelligence tactics. Once again a formidable foe since the cold war. This new inner space race could prove to be the most challenging battleground yet.

The defense department issued a full scale alert and lock down of several airports and ports in lieu of the president's presence. The first lady was handed the keys to the kingdom in the interim, pending safe return of her husband a mere 45 minutes hence.

A total 'lockdown'? It could cause mass panic and hysteria. They certainly couldn't stop what they couldn't see. But to declare a state of national emergency at the drop of a hat or former Russian agent unthinkable. She paced nervously around the room. They required the first lady's signature in his absence to abdicate her husband's reign. She had to maintain her composure and rule over her loyal subjects. It may soon rain rockets from Russia or an infinite number of sources she feared. Her imagination ran amuck. Slowly she reigned in her emotions, and decided what to do.

In one of the world's largest harbors at Hampton Roads in N. Virginia, just east of the nation's capitol. Chesapeake Bay lay about 200 km down the Potomac. A veritable waterway past the front steps of the Whitehouse. A group of wide eyed tourists lapped up the learned tour guides pearls. They realized the region was steeped in history as they huddled around him, continuing to expel numerous snippets of trivia.

"Off shore one of the most vicious battles of the civil war took place between the Confederate forces, CSS Merrimack and the Union vessel the USS Monitor. Essentially 'floating batteries',"
A few kids ruminated over the misinterpretation, a clever invention, if only batteries could float?
"..uh gunboats, ended in a stalemate. But the boats were no match for the mighty ironclads." The crowd captivated and in awe of the natural beauty, took a deep breath. Bombarded by the sordid shenanigans of their American ancestors, they awaited the next round of data. The tour guide led them to large models, replicas of the vessels and entire alignment of the fleet at the time of the stand off. In the background, the picturesque natural port

hosted a small flotilla of fishing vessels and pleasure craft as they passed through a narrow constriction past Hamptons. It wove it's way into the inner waterway toward Washington. The Potomac practically led right past the Whitehouse. A few fisherman tied their bait around their colorful lures then pointed in the general direction of the capitol. The captain cast off and let out a significant length of fishing line. Satisfied with his toss, he concurred,

"The really big ones are further upstream" he chuckled, the crew caught off guard by the off the cuff remark. Had he meant the fish? Or the high ranking government officials? No matter, it was a perfect day. They didn't want to let petty politics interfere with their outing. They wished only a few of the select senators a swift ousting as they shuffled through their tackle.

From a payphone somewhere in the metro DC district, a medium build tourist clad in typical jeans and baseball cap attire prior to a Nationals home game placed a local call.

Another tourist rushed across their hotel room to answer their cell phone.

"All aboard?" asked the curious excited citizen.

Impossible to determine their country or city of origin, now a member of the massive melting pot,

"Slipped in like a charm. No more noticeable than mote in their eyes" said the elusive raspy voice on the other end of the line. The mixed coded message came through loud and clear. Mote referring to 'smart dust' or MEMS, microelectro-mechanical sensors; wireless radio controlled devices much like the small toy sailboats at the water's edge, about the size of a grain of sand. To communicate, sense, similar to the ones installed inside the Proteus and similar devices developed by the CMDF. Practically impossible to detect, yet a highly effective way to carry out the desired task.

At Reagan airport arrivals, on the south side of the Potomac, serving greater DC and surrounding area, several passengers were patted down and scanned. Security was instantly escalated following the unsubstantiated and to some far fetched sci fi claims by the Russian agent. Nevertheless, no stone remained unturned in the intense sifting process that ensued. Easier for a camel to pass through the eye of a needle said a few airport checkers presumptuously rushing passengers through the full body scanners.

A white Caucasian of eastern European descent passed through the radiation, and micro particle scanner to detect the emission of explosive molecular particulate matter then stepped up to the counter. The passenger with a thick heavy Russian accent fished through his papers in his briefcase for his passport. The excessive radiation levels tipped off the security. They took him to a secure holding area for further questioning. They urged he take a seat. He complied, grateful to take a load off his feet.

"You ever been to Archangelsk recently?" they questioned. Reluctantly or from a faulty memory or simply a game of charades the passenger replied,

"No" he laughed lying through his teeth. Were they mocking him, as they took a cheap shot below the belt about the state of disarray of the rusting relics of their nuclear fleet. Why, even the citizens had ridiculed the Russian government about the free medical services offered 'free x-rays', from the highly radioactive emissions. In a flashback, he drifted off, prompted by the jet lag or by the sheer volume of operative memories clouding his brain into the GRU (Glavnoye Razvedyvatel'noye Upravleniye) headquarters, a younger , robust variant of the worn down operative.

The Russian Federation of Armed Forces, a mirror image of the American CMDF or Counter Miniaturization Deterrent Forces network. Who was in charge the rebels or the Russian military? The guest, a high ranking counterintelligence agent was escorted to a golf cart sized maglev vehicle full of GRU and KGB agents. They were quickly whisked down the long narrow passageway toward a check point. They pressed their faces against a padded console as the retinal scanner verified their authenticity. Coupled with a confirmed fingerprint pattern, the large vault allowed their entrance.

"Colonel Gorbikev."

"Da."

"Welcome, we have a 'small' token of appreciation for you" stated the commander of the GRU as he steered the golf cart into the busy beehive of activity. The apprehensive agent shook the hands of the top military brass. He had heard of the facility, but wasn't sure of the extent of scientific experimentation conducted there. He was led to a counter. A sleek smooth leather briefcase sat, open upright. The commander slipped a baseball and a large bottle of vodka into it. The agent noticed the baseball was signed. The commander then closed the attaché case, locked it and gently placed it in the center of a series of concentric rings. A rather odd ornate tile work on the floor for such an otherwise austere work place. He was quickly escorted from the room up a set of stairs into a large computer room. It resembled the CMDF in Washington to a tee, down to the cloned computer manufacturers. Two scientists positioned the briefcase on top of a large semi spherical glass or plastic doggy dish in the cross hairs of the bull's eye then quickly left the target area. The agent waited and watched with baited breath. Expecting an explosion or new advanced laser to slice the attaché in two.

"Begin" stated the commander and nodded his head. A number of scientists activated an array of switches in sequential order. The room lit up like the stage lights at a Bolshoi ballet. The agent watched in awe as the attaché and dish began to shrink from view. An optical illusion? a clever stage trick? A sleight of hand? he mused. In seconds it disappeared completely. Next, a hexagonal podium raised from directly below the missing paraphernalia. Two security guards escorted the agent and commander back into to the enchanting enclave. What other tricks had GRU up their sleeves wondered the mystified former KGB spy. The agent noticed a nifty new way to protect his ID perhaps glancing at the small glass 'contact lens'? certainly the most sophisticated lens crafter he had ever seen. Not your ordinary optometrist's operation. Yet convinced it was no more part of his disguise to infiltrate the impenetrable perimeter of the American defenses. A scientist wearing sterile latex exam gloves hurriedly fitted the former KGB spy with his new slim ocular contact lens. They pressed it against his moist cornea. A tear of gratitude welled up in the agent's eye for no apparent reason as he replied,

"I'm touched" that they had gone to such a

great length to protect his identity. He blinked a few times and wiped a tear from his eye. If only he knew. The shrunken nuclear device now in place for a smooth transfer to an undisclosed American facility. Had the Russkies not only stolen the technology but enhanced its performance? extending their devious pleasure? Upped the ante and intermittent micromolecular elapsed time? to an unimaginable number of hours? Only time would tell.

In a special Aeroflot flight filled with countless international delegates including a contingent of top ranking Russian officials, a shapely stewardess placed a glass on a napkin with a stiff vodka, in fact a black Russian.

"Spaciba" stated the agent. He examined the dazzling kaleidoscopic reflection off the ice cubes. The contact lens had not only cleverly disguised his eye but improved his vision. He took a long swig then set the glass down and scanned the Washington Post placed on his tray. Most of the other businessmen and delegates were discussing the recent developments in the capitol. The sudden surge and rise in suspicion of foreigners entering the country was at an all time high. With the recent ridiculous scare about the missing 'briefcase nukes', he had to chuckle. Right under their very or rather above his nose. A brave nuke or new era after the cold war was about to commence. He tested the peripheral vision of the impediment in his eye, by peering out the airliners large oval window; a beautiful panorama of Washington DC. Slightly obscured, cloudy, the bustling naval yards nearby, vessels moored along the Potomac. He zoomed in on the Washington monument as the pilot had to circle about the cloud bank and renegotiate a final approach. He spotted the state capitol and White House and the mall, a plethora of massive buildings, the Aerospace and a number of historic museums. Crowds of people filled the pedestrian walkways,all about to be drastically rearranged and literally disappear in 'the wink of an eye'.

The delegates were escorted from the plane under intense secret service security and quickly rushed through customs at Reagan International airport. All just in time for the first of a busy work agenda with top senators including the president.

His recent disappearance may put a damper on some of their plans, but didn't seem to bother the GRU agent. He approached the custom's office. His passport stamped multiple times, well traveled, impressed the custom's officials.

"Nothing to declare?" asked the officer. He'd spotted the vodka bottle clearly marked duty free. A deceptive clever fake?

"No, that's for medicinal purposes. It's from duty free." The security let it go and chuckled. He had nothing to fear, DC's water was safe to drink unlike their neighbor to the south. Better safe than sorry, and mitigate a bout with Montezuma's revenge should he decide to continue galavanting around the globe.

"Nature of your stay?" he eyed his cautiously, noting his posture and any facial gestures or flinches. The custom's officer was especially trained in body language and facial ambiguities. Length of your stay?"

"Business…in…definitely" declared the bold faced operative. He'd maintained a perfect poker face. He hurried through the checkpoint after the custom's officer handed him his passport. In lieu of the lengthy inconvenience of waiting for any carry on luggage he left the building. The clock was ticking. He had to hurry. The GRU operative stepped to the curb at arrivals and hailed a cab. The impatient taxi driver drove off trying to fill or exceed his quota for the day. Impatiently he asked the fare for a destination. The passenger seemed disoriented, bewildered by coming to America or the incessant traffic. The cabby waited…as he wove in and out of traffic taking the scenic route along the Potomac.

"Pull over" stated his flustered fare. He appeared drunk and disheveled or sea sick. The GRU agent reached into his brief case and pulled the 26 oz bottle of vodka out. The cabby eyed his fare carefully, noticeably rattled, fleeing from the law? About to make a break for it, evade the fare? Even somewhat suicidal he thought. The poor guy had probably taken a beating on the stock market, about to drown his sorrows as he noticed him heave the bottle of vodka up to his face. He stood there motionless as if about to take a swig or a pee. Perhaps unaware of American state park highway and byway laws.

"Hey buddy, you can't take a pee or toss your empties into the Potomac! This is America!" shouted the cabby about to enforce his citizen's rights and make an arrest. Before he could jump from the yellow cab, the agent flung the bottle over his head. Neither a Molotov cocktail, nor even a 'message in a bottle' or empty. It tumbled head over heels toward the bank of the broad river, then nearly shattered into a million pieces as it hit the surface. It slowly meandered amongst the rocks bound to be a smash and real nuisance to city clean up crews.

"Old habits die hard" he insisted. It left little doubt, the boozer was trying to kick the habit that affected so many Russians. The fare watched the bottle float away, then took note of the time. He had to hurry. "What were you going to do, make a citizen's arrest?"

"Uh yeah" stated the stunned cabby. Undecided whether to take him aboard again, his eyes darted back and forth from the rear view mirror and the busy thoroughfare. The driver was now suspicious. The unusual behavior coupled with his disheveled drunk demeanor. He had a notion to drop him off at the local precinct, but decided not to spoil his trip his fare finally disclosed his final destination.

"The Marriot…spasiba" breathing a sigh of relief and let bygones be bygones, the cabby bolted to the target. The fare mumbled off the buildings as they approached the core as if memorized.

"Hey you taking the cabby exam?" questioned the puzzled driver.

"Da" nodded the know it all misfit.

"Well, namin' the buildings around the mall's murder" he declared recalling his own trials and tribulations of attributing a title to each of the countless structures lining the promenade from the Lincoln Memorial to the State Capitol. He wanted to point out that it was frequented by 24 million visitors a year but thought he already knew that. He crossed the Potomac bridge into Washington. On either side the agent noticed a strong American naval presence. As he pulled into the Marriot driveway, he wondered whether to alert the authorities about a whacko walking the streets of DC but refrained as he paid his fare in full and them some. Decidedly down on his luck. A shower, shave and short reprieve may get the foreigner back on his feet. The passenger disappeared amongst the businessmen rushing to their meetings and conferences in the fashionable hotel. The agent checked in at the front desk, signed the guest register and was handed his keyless entry card. He bolted from the front desk closely guarding his briefcase, never once letting it out of his grip or sight. Once inside his hotel room, he set it down and breathed a sigh of relief as he checked his Russian astronaut watch, then rushed into the ensuite to clear and wash his eyes. He studied his face in the large vanity mirror and thought to himself,

".. 'Why beholdest thou the mote that is in thy brother's eye, but considerest not the beam that is in thine own eye.'" (Matthew 7:3 KJV). He carefully plugged the basin, then removed the contact lens ever so gently and set it onto the counter. His heart pounding, he raced to the small mini fridge by the wet bar and cracked the seals on several small vodka shot bottles. He ripped the paper wrapper from the complementary glass and poured the contents of the bottles hurriedly into the glass and downed it.

"Ah, that hits the spot" he stated. The contact lens began to grow into an electric shaver size metal object or a cell phone. He stroked the stubble on his face, almost a day's growth. He'd aged noticeably since leaving Moscow. The object continued to expand. Ultimately it grew to the size of a laptop, or the original shiny silver metallic briefcase carrying the contents. Namely one autographed baseball, tickets to the Nationals home opener at RFK (Robert F Kennedy) formerly DC Stadium, with a 45,00 capacity crowd. He snapped the latches and examined the contents, exactly as they were restored to their original condition prior to the incredible shrinking process.

"Hasta la vista DC. Batter up! Play ball!"

6: Fill 'er Up

'There's nothing serious in mortality.
All is but toys; renown and grace is dead.
The wine of life is drawn, and the mere
Lees is left this vault to brag.'

- William Shakespeare
MacBeth II iii

The pesky operative prepared to pay his respects at the season home opener unaware of the president's present condition or whereabouts. He presumed the star statesman would be there to throw the first pitch prior to the start of the game.

A minor oversight with far reaching consequences. Certainly incapable of knowing the extent of the patient's incapacitated state of mind and body. The man, relatively relaxed and composed, from several shots of the potent elixir which went straight through the blood brain barrier. A million thoughts crossed his mind as he prepared the special delivery package that packed a such a powerful punch. A calamity of cataclysmic proportions about to be unleashed on an unwary sea of fans at the home opener. In casual attire, the cool collect counter intelligence spy left the building and headed toward the metro station only two blocks from the Whitehouse, near the national mall, connecting him to a plethora of prominent landmarks. Amongst a sea of fans and regular riders of the rapid transit tram that encompassed the nation's capitol, the man wore a baseball cap to blend in inconspicuously. His only odd accessory, one silver briefcase somewhat concealed in a back pack. The train came along right on time and screeched to a stop. The floodgates opened as a surge of sightseers left the passenger car replaced by an equal number of eager sport's fans. Filled to capacity, the train took off toward its destination. Across the river, the harbor, a safe haven for hundreds of military craft, from fast frigates to missile cruisers and gunboats. The GRU gopher counted the number of his nemeses, then chuckled. A fairly even playing field, even steven in fact. The tranquil waters were traversed by all types of advanced American vessels, including a few newer prototypes always proudly on display for all the president's men including the entire defense ministry entourage, an added placebo and sense of security. The safety net scoured the channel for any sign of suspicious or covert activity in such close proximity to the Presidential palace. Across a sweeping grand panoramic view of the Potomac, an odd piece of floating debris, a lone vodka bottle, bobbed just along the surface of the water, then drifted slowly down stream.

**

In the Whitehouse situation room the first lady and defense staff grasped the gravity of the situation debating the latest news broadcast; not a pretty picture.

"Did you hear that? They've found a way to

miniaturize molecules for more than an hour!" noted the first lady noticeably edgy. How and when did the Russians edge out the advanced American breakthrough? Obviously another successful counter coupe by the clever KBG or GRO agents. Persistently taxing the security force's patience, encryption techniques and game plans. This incident certainly the straw that broke the camel's back. Heads would roll once the perpetrators were brought to justice. Likely a long list of insiders, scientists, defectors, that probably went all the way to the top of the senatorial totem pole. She watched the flag waving outside on the grounds. Red, white and blue. Such fierce national pride. It reminded her suddenly, that indeed, the president may be detained indefinitely, missing his date with the dedicated baseball fan base, and miss a golden opportunity to redeem himself and salvage several million votes. A strong support of sports and the arts, his staff still working on a viable excuse for his unmistakable absence. A body double had been considered, but deemed too deceptive. They could even postpone the game indefinitely pending the president's speedy, steady recovery. She even prayed for a little rain. As everyone on staff knew, on each of us a little rain must fall once in a while.

"We're facing a clear and present danger! The sum of all fears" stated a defense staffer, caught up in the heat of the moment and an avid aficionado of cleverly concocted chillers by Tom Clancy, that often hit too close to home. Yet the lessons learned deemed invaluable and in terms of modifications and minor adjustment to secret service security agendas and counter measures.

"Have they slipped a brief case into the United States right under our noses?" questioned the department of defense staff riled by the Fox report. Presumptuously, arrogantly taunting the top brass, he pounded his fist defiantly on the solid oak board room table. His heart skipped a few beats it seemed as his blood was brought to the boiling point. The general feared he'd soon have to go under the knife alongside the president it they didn't find a way to releases some steam from this pressure cooker slowly simmering to a boil.

"How do we check for moles?" asked the junior joint chief of staffer, and youngest member of the select committee. He recalled from his formative days in chemistry class, the importance of adding just the right minute molecular amount of a compound to arrive at the proper mixture. Any deviation from the prescribed formula could prove catastrophic and fatal. In dermatological circles an unwanted superficial blemish of the skin. The term also encompassed in the espionage world the name for a defector or an informant. Three terms, three strikes at bat. The dire expression on the entire defense staff's faces said it all. How on earth were they to prevent penetration of the perimeter of the 3rd largest nation on earth. The daunting task of guarding entrance via land, sea or air practically impossible.

"„,not only a wall" such as the Iron Curtain? We need a bubble around America" urged the first lady as she equated the sinister 'mote' or mole with a pesky air born plague, brought in on any avian vector, human body or commercial aircraft. They shared in her grief and frustration. Yet their dismal chances at preventing such a 'plague' of epic proportions was near impossible. TSA and NSA were up to their eyeballs in eliminating any threats at the border. Yet even unwanted entry at the ports was only relieved by a few percentage points. The difference between a successful second term and utter failure now hung in the balance she feared. The party had to save face and reassure the American public the president would show up full of vim and vigor, up and at 'em inspite of all the sordid rumors circulating around the capitol and the nation.

**

In the OR, an ominous silence befell the surgical staff. An unexpected close call nearly caused a catastrophic end to the mission midstream. The nurse wiped the sweat from the brow of the surgeon before he'd even had a chance to touch a surgical scalpel. A procedure still pending as the Proteus approached the chest region. They'd narrowly evaded a vicious bout in a venous return valve.

"Could've crushed the sub like a fine Bordeaux or Napa Valley grape" exuded the captain of the Proteus. He breathed a sigh of relief after he'd negotiated the chicane type constriction. The aperture bearing down upon the submersible so fast, it caught him completely by surprise. He looked back in utter shock at the tightly wound aperture that slowly loosened up a little. Dr Mancini missed the moment of life and death deliberating over the detailed anatomical charts.

"I think I might take some time off in Napoli once this ordeal is over and sample a fine Chablis or Lacryma Christi." The grapes grew on the fertile slopes of the volcano Vesuvius near Naples. After Lucifer was expelled from heaven, it caused Christ to shed a tear which dropped down into the soil. On a more solemn note, Dr Gum recalled the lines, by Paul McCartney, about a grand old painter Picasso, 'who died last night, this is what he said to us all, drink to me drink to my health, you know I can't drink any more'. He hoped they'd all soon be roasting and toasting the resident upon a successful completion of the mission. Dr Gum noticed an odd addition to the few items the crew had brought with them. He hadn't noticed the briefcase before.

"A previous passenger leave a carry on behind?" he quipped. "Or is this your make up kit?" he asked of his pretty assistant.

"Everything you see is au naturel" stated Pam

defiantly. “Well almost everything.” She came clean as she approached the shiny carryon, her curiosity equally aroused. It certainly wasn’t aboard when they left the port. She grabbed it. It appeared much heavier than she suspected, almost impossible to move. Definitely a boat anchor or dead weight, if they needed to jettison some cargo or lighten their load in a pinch.

“Uh, that’s mine, sorry” stated Roger as he peered down from under the bubble of the crow’s nest. The crew paused, momentarily amused, then went about their tasks to prepare for their arrival in the aorta. Dr Gum began to wonder what he might’ve concealed and why. Not another counter agent or spy aboard about to jeopardize the entire mission? Even Pam became perturbed at the careless gesture.

“Sparks will fly!” she fumed, neither intending a double entendre, nor pleased with his lapse in good judgment, “…when we get to customs. You should have declared everything!” She broke out into a hearty laugh, realizing her faux pas.

“I’ll be sure to alert the authorities. You’ll be the first to know” he stated quickly without arousing any more suspicion from the crew. He downplayed the decidedly obvious and as of yet undisclosed contents to the crew. Pam peered at the object, still not convinced and pulled a hairpin from her large disheveled hair done into a bouffant ball hairdo. Her efforts proved futile as she tried to pry the cover from the carry on case. Roger smirked from atop his perch preparing for the most precarious part of the mission. About to enter the chambers of the stopped heart. A resumption of the familiar lub dub would prove fatal, if the president were to be revived for what ever reason. They'd be crushed like a grape in a winepress.

Dr Gum, like a sous chef or chemistry professor, began to stir the soupy concoction of stem cells mass manufactured especially for this mission. The mixture was then extracted from the large 'aquarium' with a squeezable pouch like that used by a pastry chef. It was placed into a 'soccer ball or breast type pump. He then inserted the gooey gumbo type broth into each bucky ball. The icing 'inside' the cake, not on top of it.

**

The presidential entourage paced nervously about

the room. Waiting for any word on the where abouts of an abandoned briefcase, particularly in the down town or metro DC area.

"What are they up to?" asked the first lady. She knew neither whence they came nor their sordid past. But the perpetrators were already amongst Americans, likely since the days of the cold war. Watching, waiting to infiltrate the very fabric of American society. She shifted her focus of attention to much more pressing imminent and presumably predictable details. "Any word on the president? I wish he were here to handle this growing crisis." Not on the scale of a full blown Cuban Missile crisis, yet, but the bewildering psycho babble by the Bolshevik betrayer left them spellbound. Merely smoke and mirrors blown out of proportions to psych out the party? Or was there much more to the madmen than met the eye? He was in the intelligence business not unlike their own CIA and CMDF counter terrorists spies. Information was the name of the game. Perhaps a coded message, yet the presence of the briefcase nukes proven to not only exist, but mishandled by the Russians themselves. Lost, stolen, found again in the most bizarre places. Why she wouldn't be surprised if one turned up on the desk in the Oval Office one day, disguised as Fuller Brush man's wares.

The joint chiefs of staff rallied around the feisty iron fisted female awaiting word on their chief. The former naval and ex nuclear sub commander was embroiled in the midst of a marine mess of epic proportions. The tide and tables turned, he was under intense naval surveillance, the likes of which he'd never dreamt of. Unfathomable a few decades back. The department of defense staff did not like the way the ducks were all aligning themselves in a row. Too close for comfort, they decided to go to yellow alert, and Defcon 3. A strike on domestic soil seemed both plausible and imminent. They alerted the USCG to go to high alert and tighten the ports along the Potomac.

"We'll catch this red herring. This pinko commie red handed!" reiterated the revered rear admiral. The red herring reference foremost on his minds. Versed in all manner of tactical diversions, he remembered the Washington Red Skins were in town to play in National park. He'd recalled the tragic turn of events in Baltimore during a Super bowl game during the fictitious film 'Sum of All Fears'. Unsettled by the sequence of events and fearing a repeat performance, he urged the defense department and detachment of the national guard to be on the look out and step up security at the game. Perhaps a little Russian roulette, and inspite of the president's slated attendance at the Washington Nationals home opener, he couldn't help but wonder what they were up to.

"But where, when…and how? A suitcase is so visible" reasoned the first lady. If only her husband were here. He'd know what to do. Yet the brunt of the bewildering almost boastful statement fell clearly on her shoulders. She now knew what it meant to walk a mile in the president's shoes. She'd likely covered that much ground pacing back and forth in the situation room by now. "I want port authority scans from here to Virginia stepped up! No container will be left unturned." Although she meant to say no stone left unturned, the port being a mere stone's throw away from the capitol, the chiefs of staff caught the drift. Each and every leisure craft gently drifting up the Potomac was meticulously checked. "Unless…"

"Unless?" asked the staff anxiously awaiting any solution to their dire dilemma.

"Oh nothing" stated the resourceful riddle and cross word puzzle solver as she pondered the inconceivable. Could the Russians have miniaturized the nuclear device? It was unheard of and hadn't crossed the minds of anyone present. She didn't want to alarm them needlessly any more than she had to. And now understood full well why the president had suffered a massive heart attack. This job was for the birds! The bewildering mountain of millions of unaddressable problems that crossed his desk daily. Inundated with life or death decisions. Why this was a job for no one less than superman or other hero bestowed with super powers! The stress could kill an army of assistants, let alone one man.

In the OR, the blip gently crossed the threshold from the aortic arch into the upper atria of the heart. Roger gently eased the submersible into the bewildering labyrinth of chordae tendinae still tensed connecting each of the valves. The only way in or out of the sequential chamber of horrors. His heart had suffered massive irreparable damage by conventional surgical standards. A complete transplant not out of the question. Yet the doctors felt the road to a full recovery was better suited by a regenerative stem cell approach. The guidance system avoided the long sinuous strands of tendons stretched between each valve like long vines or strings of a symphony orchestra. He couldn't allow the Proteus to get entangled in the myocardial mesh. Escape near impossible, pending a complete depletion of the CO2 laser, in the tethered trap other than the operating site.

**

A massive military search was mobilized. The large portable x-ray scanners were wheeled into position, parked parallel to the plethora of cargo containers entering the Virginia port authority recently from a departure point in Aden near the Middle East. The nervous crew speaking a broken scattered English shuffled nervously about the deck trying desperately to conceal something as customs security and SWAT teams stormed the vessel. They hid their weapons just as the custom's officials arrived. Drilled and grilled the translator finally coaxed them to cough up some information and answer a few questions, fast.

"Show him the picture" urged the port authority security official.

"Have you seen these? asked a veteran to the force showing him a photo of a shiny silver brief case. He'd seen every form of fake, cloned, mass produced piece of paraphernalia enter the busy thoroughfare. The Muslim man marveled the shiny apparel, nodding favorably at it's appearance. "You have these aboard?" He shrugged his shoulders then passed the photo around. The crew shook their heads defiantly, they had never seen anything like it before. They'd certainly like to knock off a few hundred, perhaps thousands, to trade on the black market, and underway on a much larger scale in Hong Kong and mainland China. Billions was lost each year to illicit counterfeiting of pilfered merchandise. Anything from CDs, DVDs, designer duds; that demanded a scrutinously meticulous inspection. The quality of cloned goods and logos became legendary.

The men pleaded their innocence as the heavily armed border patrol hurried past the perplexed crewmen. Their suspicions soon confirmed as the massive portable flat slab almost as large as the television screen inside the NFL franchise in Dallas Cowboys stadium, was rolled alongside the vessel. The eerie enhanced x-ray visual virtually verified any colonoscopies or recent dental work. It identified the chemical composition and molecular makeup of essentially everything stored or concealed on board. Lead stuffed teddy bears imported from China enroute to the mainland USA, cheap knock offs, fake jewelry were all disclosed. The items fitting the description of the photographs were definitely not aboard. One of the men received a tip in the earphone plug inserted into his baseball cap. He quickly ordered half his men to exit the ship immediately to pursue a lead else where in the vast entrance point. The FBI and NSA had been tipped off to a small fishing fleet of unknown origin coming into the channel. In the process they nabbed several rogue vessels entering via Norfolk and Hamptons. The culprits were corralled and herded off the high tech fleet of cleverly disguised fishing craft. Outfitted with the latest communication link ups to a foreign military satellite network. The stash, a large sample of extensive electronic components, sophisticated scanners and surveillance equipment, obviously not meant for NSA or FBI consumption. They planned to even the playing field by offering their partners in crime comparable tactical components to watch and listen in on the listeners.

"Listen up, we're getting very warm!" insisted the inspector.

"I dunno...." questioned the knowledgeable terrorist negotiator. "why, by the time we blink, another billion dollars worth of bogus bootlegged black market merchandize will've slipped into America."

"Fill'er up" urged the armed port authorities as they rounded up the respectable size of seized surveillance equipment. It definitely severed a vital line and chink in the chain of communication to the crooked command centers somewhere in the Middle east. One more reason to step up security and remain vigilant in the war against terror. The rate of persistent fiends penetrating and infiltrating the very fabric of civilized society continued to grow by leaps and bounds.

**

The streets of the capitol were meticulously scoured. No amount of foreign effluent remained. Inspite of a policy of non racial or ethnic profiling, a few innocent citizens were falsely accused and apprehended. If the president were present to witness the inexcusable exercise, a few heads would've rolled reasoned the resistance.

The security guards were scattered thin as they scoured the bleachers and outfield for particulate matter or particularly suspicious behavior from the fans. A futile exercise indeed. Half of the roaring crowd sat wearing their colorful ball caps, a +ve ID could take hours. To find a man matching the man description leaving the Marriot, near the Metro practically impossible. Millions fitted that description, slowly, painstakingly whittled down to tens of thousands. Security personnel scoured the locker rooms as the teams left to make a grand entrance onto the ball diamond and into the bull pen to warm up.

"Hey you, what're you doin' here?" wondered the ball park patrolman. The elusive man, presumably on the maintenance crew or janitorial staff, left in a flash. He left the lockers slightly ajar. The security guard flashed his powerful pocket light into the locker. He found a leather hard ball in the upper compartment, rolling about ever so slightly. Thinking he'd caught the thief red handed, he reached up into the space and picked up the coveted prized possession. He looked at the unusual chicken scratch yet couldn't identify it. "Got it. Got myself an autographed ball." He mulled his options. The team wouldn't mind if they misplaced a ball or two. Likely signed by one of the top batters planning to blast it out of the park. Save the lucky individual, fortunate enough to catch the pop fly, the trip back and have the home run hitter autograph it. Always thinking ahead he chuckled.

7: Play Ball

'All we can do is play ball. Every time we go out on the field, we do what we do in America, live in the freedom our country affords us.'

- Tim Salmon, former MLB great known as the 'King Fish'

He tossed the leather clad sphere up into the air. The motion detector inside, still inactive, was not tripped. The guard rolled the round relic in his sweaty palms. Likely fetch a pretty penny some day.

"Hey, let me see that. I can identify the writing" came a raspy voice out of the shadows. It was the man under question. Not on maintenance or ball park staff at all. A regular Joe, a fan? What was he doing outside the locker room? Had he tried to swipe the souvenir? He looked familiar. One of the national's sport's writers he figured. A harmless request in itself. He certainly had the ways and means to insist the inquisitive type give the ball back!

"Certainly." The guard took his stance emulating his favorite future draft pick, Steven Strasbourg? A huge strikeout potential? He wound up and rifled the ball erratically to the baseball fan who nervously caught the pitch in his cap. He wiped the sweat from his brow, then gently removed the ball from his cap. The writing was on the wall as he pulled a silencer from his pants and plugged the guard full of lead. He dragged the body into a maintenance closet and exchanged the uniform and fake ID then left the closet; the guard gagged, bound, and still out cold, covered under mops and cleaning materials. He had to hurry now, to place the ball into the press box. The forged signature by a KGB specialist looked like the real McCoy. The official 'first ball' expected to be tossed out by the president himself, already signed bearing his seal of approval. The delicate accelerometer inside, set to activate a detonator inside his portable brief case nuke to start the final countdown sequence, some where inside the capitol, perhaps even in the National Park Stadium. Such a fitting season opener, bound to begin with a bang. Coupled with the national anthem, he could already imagine the 'rocket's red glare… and the bombs bursting in air'…He assumed a full retaliatory strike in the event of the cleverly orchestrated plan going off without a hitch! The guard picked up his pace as he arrived at the press box, then peered out over the infield. 45,000 fans vaporized in the wink of an eye. It didn't seem to phase him. He simply wanted to insure that he 'pitch his proposal' properly. He'd only have one crack at it he reasoned approaching the radio host and inquired where to drop off the ball for the president. The radio announcer assumed in the 'dugout', where the secret service intended to whisk the leader of the free world to pick up the leather clad orb to toss the first pitch and urge the teams to 'play ball!

**

The defense staff shuffled about, congratulating one another with a solid handshake. An aging relic, and retired rear admiral clipped the end off a Cuban stogy and lit it. The premature celebration if only a brief pause, and a positive placebo following the recent raid on the docks. The determined effort had reeled in only a few of the smaller fish, the feisty relentless rebel resistors determined to deliver a message loud and clear. The cleverly concealed communication's components caught just in the nick of time. The staff passed their praises generously around the room, pleased with the progress to sever the life line linking the lethal operatives still on the loose. Their financial life boats of support deflated, their ties to known terrorist havens in their holy land severed.

"We're close, but still no cigar" fretted the first lady softly. The smoke irritated her eyes yet did not state her displeasure, allowing the indulgence for a job well done. So many docks, so little time to intervene. Where and when they'd strike next? and what on earth the agent referred to, still a complete mystery. She had a notion to bring the braggart into custody if only to clarify what his presumptuous claims were all about. Fox hadn't a clue, other than the brief broadcast to cause quite a stir on the countless television screens in the state capitol, let alone the nation. The cheap trick harped on the horrendous financial and psychological impact of the direct hit on American soil within the past decade. It appeared to work, playing on the psyche of the people creating a general sense of unease and elevated suspicion amongst the citizens. The only palliative measure, to take their minds off the madmen, and go out to the old ball game, with a box of cracker jacks and a hot dog and 'play ball'. It was the American way. Nothing would dampen the spirits and resolve of the serious sports enthusiasts. The rest resided in the hands of the top NSA dogs scouring the docks. The men armed with sniffer dogs quickly caught the scent of more suspicious sordid nefarious activities. It all led down blind alleys and wild goose chases, albeit a sizeable amount of weaponry was confiscated in counterfeit eider down feather pillows just pulling into port. All roads seemed to lead to Washington. The time and place of the next strike imminent in the immediate vicinity sensed the commander in chief in her husband's absence. The smoke began to bother her.

"Those things'll kill you" she commented, subtly requesting the rear admiral butt out. He paused momentarily to mull at the only lady present then blew a loud ring of smoke across the room defiantly. It dissipated on the virtual map of the Metro DC area and quickly radiated from the center of the map, near the NW sector of the city approximately where Bethesda naval facility lay. Her husband somewhere several multiple stories below the surface. Her subconscious seemed to kick into overdrive, the wheels turning. It was high time for them to seek the shelter of the White House bunker, to survive an imminent nuclear strike. She could feel it in her bones. "Why, one of those smoke particles and specks of dust or pollen could carry a concealed miniaturized nuke into the country." She thought about the ridiculousness of her statement. Yet factoring in all the fictitious notions that had become science fact, it wasn't so far fetched. Her husband inconceivably under intense investigation by a naval vessel inside his circulatory system a case in point. 40 years ago, the mere mention of nano technology the subject of sheer sci fi speculation on the silver screen. Now a proven reality and respected remedy. 'Imagination is infinitely more important than knowledge' harped Einstein often. The woman knew it best to soon make a move to a safer location under the hallowed grounds. Better safe than sorry. Several more reports in rapid succession were relayed to the Whitehouse. The unprecedented chatter left little to the imagination. A clear and present danger on American soil existed. The generals quickly responded.

"Take us down to Defcon 2." Defcon 1 now a distinct possibility. The secret service staff were ready to escort the top brass and bolt to the bunker at a moment's notice. The generals tried to think like the cunning terrorists, and predict their intended targets. Try as they might, they could not assume or ascertain their modus operandi. All major venues were in a state of near lockdown. The opera, the theaters, the countless cultural events. All indications were the fiends had found a favorable 'nest'. The Nuclear Emergency Support Teams under the direction of the Nuclear National Security Administration were standing by. The committee had calculated the extent of a lethal cloud of radioactive particulate matter that may soon encompass the capitol. Casualties from a catastrophic nuclear blast could climb into the millions. The best case scenario, a small briefcase nuke carrying a dirty bomb or biohazard weapon, limited by it's location, shielded in the subway, or a shelter. Mitigating a massive head count; EMS and all available hospitals in a STAT state. Escape routes impossible to determine at this juncture. Reagan Airport on imminent lockdown, standing by to whisk the White house staff away in Air Force one to a safe location in a neighboring state. And to send a NEST response team consisting of a few helicopters and planes outfitted with sensitive detection technology in ASAP. The prominent naval presence along the Potomac also in imminent and present danger. A few of the newest fastest frigates able to encapsulate their crew in a hermetically sealed shell. Serving as the first line of defense and responders in the event of a colossal calamity. The hot zone difficult to maneuver and initiate emergency medical response as the analysts and strategists could only imagine from all the simulated exercises. The teams were still sifting through visible accessories fitting the description of the briefcase. All businessmen had returned to the sanctity of their homes following the afternoon rush, radically reducing the random raids on offices. The eager beavers, late or all night computer geeks and software staff the first to be preyed upon. Their briefcases and back packs open, crammed with circuits and chips, and munchies. Neither the citizens pleased by the sudden unexpected surprise 'visits' by the NSA and local authorities. Several helicopters suddenly swooped down on unsuspecting businessmen crossing the bridge into Washington. The bright floodlights nearly forced them to flee and jump for their lives from the bridge, utterly mystified by the precautionary measure. The men mistaken, lumped in with all the lethal terrorists, their attaches by their sides, considered highly suspicious, by the cautious pilot and copilots.

A wave of elevated arms rapidly traversed National Park stadium near the heart of Washington. The restless fans sought their illustrious commander in chief. The avid baseball fanatic was fashionably late. The late arrival allowed the scalpers to skin a measurable amount of mullah from the desperados seeking seats. Expecting a packed house, standing room only and nosebleed sections also sold out. The boisterous bravado of the concerned loyal fan base cloaked the relative credibility of a bomb threat. They cheered noisily and urged the man of the hour to make a fast and furious appearance.

"No sign of the president yet?" noted the anxious park officials. They were waiting patiently for the familiar armored motorcade. No where in sight nor given the head's up by any of the white house staffers, a typical brief in the chain of command. They grew concerned that something wasn't quite right. A no show, so out of character for the charismatic leader. Had the entourage already been tipped off to a potentially catastrophic tragedy before the onset of the home opener? The press section dispelled any suspected no show with a brief vote of confidence of their own.

" 'Fraid not. He's never missed a season opener." They spilled the beans. The restless rambunctious crowd about to go into riot mode, sought an immediate response or reasonable explanation for his absence. In any event they knew 'the show must go on' and urged the umpire to beckon the ball players onto the field to 'play ball!'

Mayhem moment's away, several scalpers and senseless fans climbed the perimeter fences if only to catch a glimpse of president Taylor. Ethnic groups of all flavors flooded the fences. It brought a whole new meaning to the opening anthem, 'Jose can you see?...by the dawn's early light.' Neither Jose climbing the interlinking metal mesh, nor any other spectator was able to witness the world leader now likely a no show before the crack of dawn as the minutes turned to half an hour.

**

"Time?" asked the CMDF commander lost in deep thought. The giant atomic clock loomed ominously right in front of his face. The monitors and president's vitals stable, purring along perfectly. The patient pleasantly perfused with sedatives and blood thinners, like the 'boy in a bubble'. Hermetically sealed in his own private little universe far removed from the maddening crowd. Totally at the mercy of the Maquet heart lung machine and the talented men and women waiting for the minute by minute progress report of the crew. Tethered to the plastic lifeline delivering the oxygenated liquid, a delicate balancing act, to replenish the life saving solution. The dark red deoxygenated blood quickly evacuated into the labyrinth of rollers and pumps then returned, rejuvenating the patient, resting peacefully, everything going perfectly according to plan.

The rest lay in the hands of the four crew of the curious little submersible craft slowly closing in on the target. The sub slowly slipped into the final few turns on the home stretch to the scarred tissue. The blue deoxygenated depleted RBC supply a sign they were still on course.

"Somewhere down the crazy river…catch the blue stream…" Roger paused to ponder how far they had come. Not only the crew but all of mankind. The marvelous working of the human mind. Second only to the human heart. Without its relentless merciless maintenance of the meandering river of life, our very thoughts and actions a mere mirage. Impossible without the very essence or sustenance of the circulatory system. They were only guests here, granted a brief glimpse to witness the grandeur and vast scope of God's universe seen by few eyes. "To places never seen before." (Robby Robertson lyrics) .

The tiny blip, still burning brightly, signifying a symbol of hope for the prostrate patient resting in peace, and the crew still very much alive and intact crossed a threshold into the heart.

"They're inside. They'll have 30 minutes to 'operate'. God speed." His reference to the vessel bearing the same name, 'Godspeed', one of captain Newport's three ships at the 1st landing near Virginia Beach in 1607 no mere coincidence. He only hoped they'd reached the distant shore of the scarred heart tissue in similar good spirits.

"We're in the right atrium" stated Dr Mancini comparing his medical expertise in performing countless open heart surgeries to the monstrous landscape looming outside. The thick tangled mesh like the blue bayou foliage or tropical rainforest hung from the top of the voluminous vault to the floor of the caves like overextended stalagmites and stalactites. A veritable paradise for any spelunker or deep sea diver lay before his eyes.

"It looks like Swiss Cheese" postulated Pam, the only culinary reference point she could think of. The void in the pit of her stomach prompted her to think of only a favorite food time. Coupled with a tasty palate thirst quencher, a Chablis or Reisling, a fitting finale to a job hopefully well done.

"We'll avoid the IVC, one of our potential escape routes" insisted Sparks, plotting his course carefully and not overshoot the intended target. The sub inched toward the small slit in a sluggish sea of pooled blood residing in the vast reservoir.

"That way, through the tricuspid valve" stated Mancini as he established the nature of the unique tripartite opening in the wall outside the view port. Their 'window of opportunity', a hazardous trap during normal operation of the marvelous pump, open sufficiently to allow access to the president's very private inner sanctum.

"Language is the blood of the soul into which thoughts run and out of which they grow"

(Oliver Wendell Holmes Sr., American professor, lecturer, author) said the startled dentist. His cardiac surgical colleagues had always suggested he switched to their specialty. Now he knew what they meant marveling the unbelievable labyrinth. He commented on the seat of the soul and their inevitable departure before the hour was up or become one with the president in the most peculiar way. Their imminent logarithmic growth in size of considerable concern concurred the heart specialist. Macrophages and all manner of defense systems would kick in at that time and insure they leave before they'd outlived their welcome. The right auricle a tangled spider web, waiting to capture and ensnare its prey. The sub foremost on the endangered species list. There was some evidence of bacterial endocarditis, or prominent plaque plastered onto the walls of the tendons; an obvious sign of over indulgence and possible a recent infection. Even from a dental procedure feared Dr Gum. Text book photos paled in comparison to the ramifications found in situ.

"A mind filled with peace, creates a heart filled with contentment" remarked Sparks. The tell tale signs of the persistent stress and pressure which the president was under clearly depicted right before their eyes.

"Then why is he all jammed up? His body looks like a temple where junk food goes to worship" said Pam as she offered her two cents worth. A little common sense could have avoided the sticky wicket they were now very much a part of. Not out of the woods or thick of things by any stretch of the imagination. Sparks hoped the chorda tendinae tethered tightly held their anchorage. A sudden release of a tightly strung chord could smash the windshield and cause a catastrophic implosion.

"A ticking time bomb" noted the renown heart specialist. The evidence and writing clearly on the walls of the badly battered and bruised bacteria laden heart muscle. The erratic grey patches of necrotic scar tissue the prime targets. There was so much of it as he cringed. He realized they may have underestimated the extent of the initial infarct. The massive patchwork of plaque placed the damage at one of a lengthy accumulation of mini heart attacks contributing to the row upon row of wretched seemingly irreparable furrows. They certainly had their work cut out for them. Time was of the essence if they were to complete their mission and still have time to negotiate a safe and speedy departure. The team prepared to suit up and seek out the best angle of attack. The precious seconds ticked away. Dr Mancini and Sparks thought it best not to worry the outside world needlessly of the recent discovery. The severe ramifications might jeopardize the entire mission. The word was mum. Their lips were sealed as their wet suits soon were, the crew donned their scuba gear and entered the hatch. Armed with the CO2 laser and a few 'soccer balls' stuffed to the brim like a thanksgiving turkey, they entered the air lock. Bearing good tidings and gifts from afar, they embraced the eerie thought of touching upon this new untouched territory like time or space travelers in this strange yet wonderful world. They slowly cautiously disembarked the submersible as if severing the umbilical chord during the miracle of birth. Each now free floating in the foreign medium, like the ether of space. The current considerably stronger than it appeared from inside the vessel. There was a distinct drift, a lateral shift to the large aperture, sucking the solution toward either the SVC or IVC and out into the tubing leading into the heart lung machine.

8: Message

'Every child comes with the message that God is not yet discouraged of man.'

- Rabinadrath Tagore, Indian polymath, 1st Asian Novel Prize in Literature recipient

"Hey look, a message in a bottle!" noted one of three startled youths as they raced along the nature trails on the banks of the harbor near Hampton Roads.

"From pirates?" questioned the youngest of the three. The pop quiz likely had several possible answers they figured as they approached the rocky shore. Careful not to get their new sneakers wet as they negotiated the slippery slimy rocks.

"Pirates in America?" said the eldest of the three. He wanted to dispel the myth, but knew the harbor was often frequented by many foreign vessels. Many of whom were not even included in the pages of Jane's Fighting Ships. "Maybe it's from the 'Big Mac'?" He meant the Merrimack , the former glorious iron side, but his stomach growled, tending to the more modern variant of the phrase and it was getting close to dinner time. The tired youths decided it was definitely time to turn back before they'd get a scolding. The inquisitive teen ager crouched down and reached out to the bottle, careful not to fall in. He didn't recognize it as a clear vodka bottle, focusing on the message inside it. The teen made a few waves which allowed it to reach his outstretched fingertips. He pulled the peculiar bottle, not like the other long necked green or brown coke bottles he was familiar with, and popped the cork. Then using a slender fresh twig to try to tease the rolled note from the narrow neck of the bottle, he turned the bottle upside down topsy turvy. It proved as difficult as getting the ketchup out of a bottle of the best Heinz. Finally the note fell out. The three youths waited with baited breath as the lad unfurled the unusual but legible font.

"I'm going to make the president an offer he can't refuse'…signed Grrrrr.." he thought for a moment. Tony the Tiger? But quickly dispelled the author to an unknown.. GRU? "grew?" who knew? No one had ever heard of him. Perhaps three initials, Graham, Reginald Unger. Jim Unger, the creator of the 'Herman' comic strip or 'Herman Munster', he couldn't remember which was which; a distant relative? They'd have to let their parents check the ancestry registry when they got home.

"What does it mean?"

"I dunno. Must be one angry dude." He equated the grrrr as a menacing growl from an animal or madman, like the wolfman or Cujo. "Better ask your mom. Come on we better not be late for dinner."

He emptied the contents out into the river, then placed the unusual bottle into his back pack. The impatient boy scouts then hurried back along the windy nature trail past Willoughby Spit and Sewell Pt. where the battle of Hampton Roads had taken place near the 'Great Dismal Swamp', one of the last large pristine wild areas in the United States. The place where 7 cities converged on a near 'ice free' waterway year round. The perfect playground to the Navy, USCG, military, NASA, and even enemy craft!

The boys rushed home relieved they arrived in the nick of time. They tossed their things aside and hurried to wash up before dinner. Their pet dog instantly aroused, his curiosity piqued by the odd item sticking out of the backpack clawed at the contents. He dragged the bottle from the pack then proceeded to chew on the cork, exposing his canine menacingly. The boys towel dried their hands then hustled to the table. One of the boy's fathers noticed the perturbed demeanor of the family pet. He wondered what had gotten into Rex.

"What is it boy? What have you got there? Let me see."

The floppy eared cocker spaniel relinquished his grip on the cork spitting out the tattered chunks yet continued to bark at the bottle. The father, a veteran sheriff with the local county was equally intrigued by the resilient vodka bottle. From where and why they'd carted it home was beyond him. It was bad enough keeping the trails clear of all the plastic bottles simply tossed at the side of the pristine park area. At the current pace, future generations may not appreciate the simpler pleasures of the peaceful woodlands. Why, Americans spent more on water bottles in 2006 than I pods and movie tickets alone. $15 billion, more than 1 billion bottles per week in the US while 1/6 of the world had no fresh drinking water at all. How ironic he thought. Land of the free water, home of the brave bottlers. He tapped on the bottom of the bottle until the contents slowly plopped onto the floor. He snatched the note ere Rex ripped it apart then unfurled it like the Dead Sea Scrolls and perused the simple phrase. Perturbed at the ominous warning he put two and two together, recalling the recent Fox updates on the news. Puzzled and equally concerned he called the port authority regarding the discovery.

Eddie's father described the contents and composition and physical features of the bottle.

Where they had found it, surprisingly it had washed ashore. The brand of bottle, Stolichnaya Elit, the most expensive, around $60 USD per bottle found rarely in any of the liquor stores or even special order items, yet heavily advertised even behind home plate at New York Yankees televised games. The staple in this neck of the woods, JD - Jack Daniels, JW - Johnny Walker and the favorite, Cutty Sark, named after the seafaring vessel.

"Weel done" said the crusty old sea captain, and now port authority antique. Oft denounced, he kept his haven ship shape glad he was given the head's up. In the local pecking order, the message in a bottle quickly found its way up the chain of command all the way to the White House. The ominous note, noteworthy in itself. Not your typical disgruntled citizen, the forensics dept soon discovered a distinct match in the handwriting to those of a former defector of the KGB, now working for GRU. He must've gone to great lengths to drop the bottle off. A few statisticians reasoned it was simply a coincidence merely washing ashore near Washington, a random occurrence, the odds remote. The White House took a proactive approach. Anything that menacing was not taken lightly not left any margin for error.

"Yes thank you. We'll get on it right away." Her gut instinct told the first lady not to overlook this sign. "It's the Coast Guard. It appears we have a growing concern on our hands." The timing ticked her off. The Proteus had entered the critical juncture of the operation and passed into the president's heart chamber. More than mere coincidence? She mused. Was she and the defense staff reading too much into the discovery? Seeing what they did not want to and dreaded to see. The stars and sequence of events aligning themselves into some sort of clandestine plan. A catastrophic event they were unable to impede?

The port authority found the daunting task too time consuming. To come up with any quick fixes or answers, they worked round the clock counting, meticulously x raying and scanning every container from Timbuctoo to Tibet that came into Hampton Roads port.

"It's a lost cause" stated a weary security dock worker.

Had the bottle simply washed in with the tide? Tossed off a senator's or foreign dignitary's yacht during a midnight cruise? The region formerly known as 'tidewater', a productive tobacco growing area, set just above the 'fall line', where the rapids and waterfalls ended transitioning into the foothills. Countless slaves were brought to work in the area, at its peak almost ¾ of the house holds harbored slaves.

A group of fishermen tending their nets chuckled, sorting through their tackle, amused by the reports of a Russkie rebellion or sneak attack up the back woods. A strong USCG contingent, followed by fast frigates, a few gunboats and missile cruisers set them at ease. The strong American military presence made their task so much easier. Yet they still had their work cut out for them. The fish wouldn't find their way on board by themselves.

"Big brother's made it perfectly clear who's boss" stated the crusty former Cape Codder as he prepared to toss his line over the gunnel. The heightened state of alert coupled with a constant concern of a sneaky 'special delivery' brought an abrupt about face in formalities. The fishermen were startled by the sudden invasion of their personal space as they peered down the barrel of the cannon aboard the bow of a fast frigate. The vessel prepared to board. No craft, dinghy or stone remained unturned in the seemingly senseless search that bordered on over kill. They realized the naval vessel could alleviate a lot of needless grief and waiting time by simply depositing a depth charge in the water and send the species of fish to the surface. They thought they better not press their luck as a patrol party boarded their vessel. He dropped his lure in the process and showed their fishing permits. The search patrol scoured the small aging craft. The wretched stench of fish entrails caused the customs agents to hurl their hot breakfasts. Relieved from coming up empty handed by their random routine search they returned to their vessel. Their daily tedium so rudely interrupted, the fishermen soon resumed their daily ritual and waited with baited breath for the first nibble.

The White House staff received wind of any and all leads bombarding the building's air waves.

Anything from verified Fox reports to visually impaired citizens sensing anything suspicious. A major breakthrough came suddenly as a freighter coming in from the Middle East via the Cape of Good Hope was apprehended. The Mediterranean the shorter, preferred route, now adays, to the long way around.

"We found similar 'suitcases' to the one that fit the description of the item in question. Onboard a vessel registered in Aden, a known Al Qaeda transfer point." Pleased with the perceptive USCG's performance, not only intercepting a mass knock off of merchandise presumably for future ops, but located the manufacturer at the point of departure as well. Trouble in the air, definitely a brewin'. They seemed to let down their guard for a split second. Presumptuous? Premature celebration in the cautious censorship of incoming containers?

"We're getting awfully warm" warned the first lady. Her seasoned senses were tingling. Some thing did not sit well with her or feel right. For the first time she knew exactly what it was like to walk a mile in her husband's shoes. Her exemplary take charge attitude brought a subtle silence to the room. Her confidence and charm hopefully spread like a brush fire as did her husband's.

"Yes, thank you, keep up the good work." She appreciated the expediency and swift seizure of the goods, the communication network second to none. She was in the loop every step of the way. Playing a vital part in the country's well being and welfare. Had they nipped this thing in the bud?

Overhead, above the blinding floodlights that lit up the night sly like the 4th of July, a squadron of JSF 35 Lightning II's were just completing their rounds and returning to Joint Base Andrews Air facility 10 miles south east of Washington, DC. Camp Springs Maryland lay adjacent to the AFB. Air Force One of the 89th AV wing, was located there. The 316th wing, bestowed with the task of emergency rotor relief and evacuation contingency support. National security, training, deployment & readiness of AEFs Air and Space Expeditionary Forces.

The pilots decided to make one more pass over National Park Stadium, a clean sweep that appeared more like a formal fly by by the fly boys breaking rank with the rest of the fighter squadron formation. One for the Gipper? Referring to Ronald Reagan only in the movies. The name actually belonged to George Gipp. Planning to pursue a career in baseball, the legendary coach Knute Rockne persuaded him to play football instead. Leading the Fighting Irish to an unprecedented 27-2-3 record, many of the records still stood. His short career came to an abrupt and tragic end as he caught a throat infection and died at the young age of 25. Reagan played the Gipper in the 1940 film.

"You figure we'll see some fireworks tonight?" asked the lead pilot innocently.

"Season opener tonight isn't it?" asked the copilot as they perused the packed house. They expected to see the bases loaded or watch a pop fly to the outfield. Instead it was surprisingly quiet on the infield, the teams still stuck in suspended animation in their dugouts. The president decidedly a no show sensed the home town fans.

"Eagle eye to base over."

Joint Base Andrews Air Facility was on high alert.

"This is base. Over."

"Clear skies smiling at me. You outta get a load of this twinkling starlight" he stated citing the star studded lineup in lieu of the bright city and traffic lights sequestering most of the celestial bodies above.

"Get your butts back here. You're not on a safari sight seeing mission." With the forces spread so thin, every experienced top gun for hire served a double tour of duty. They had to fly the friendly skies 24/7 lately to provide cover if only a placebo and false sense of security.

"Roger that. Eagle eye over and out, returning to base."

Several squadrons of the 11th wing had taken off from the NCR - National Capitol Region at Andrews. Bolling AFB the former AFB directly in DC now mere ceremonial support to the president, the joint chiefs of staff. The only remaining launch pad a 100' x 100' helipad.

"I don't like it. All that chatter, then …nothing" noted a seasoned squadron leader.

"Sounds of silence gettin' to ya cap?" quipped his copilot.

"Yeah." He didn't like it one bit. The calm before

the storm sensation caused a chill as he peered out over the capitol. The excitement in the baseball stadium temporarily extinguished as everyone began to sense the man of the hour would not appear.

The pilots perused the busy metro stations, whisking the citizens to and fro from the DOT offices along the well traveled arteries countless times daily. A few late arrivals got off near the stadium hopeful and anxious to scalp a few tickets. The last minute attendees underwent scrutinous body scans and security checks, patted down, coupled with full body x-rays. A suspicious back pack was checked, impervious to penetration by the x rays. The guards quickly asked the fan to drop it for a thorough search. A 'nuclear device'? The guards grew apprehensive attempting to open it. Caught between a rock and a hard place, they paused and pondered their next move. Call in a SWAT team, the bomb squad and a robot or demolition's expert to assist in probing the pesky pack that refused to reveal its contents. Several stunned fans cleared the perimeter fearing a fatal repercussion, the Fox news reports still foremost their minds. The robot arrived shortly after being summoned. It proceeded with extreme caution. The players still warming up in the dugout, were unaware of the situation brewing outside the bleachers. They were swinging multiple bats, chewing then spitting mouthfuls of the strong tobacco onto the dusty dugout floor or into the thick green turf on the field. The pitchers rolled a few balls in their palms nervously, their knuckles poised. They cracked them a few times to ride out the endless waiting game. The fans peered out onto the field getting antsy about president Taylor's arrival. Oh where oh where could he be? Caught in traffic? Presidential motorcade problems? The unlikely odds of such an occurrence impeding his presence a million or more to one. The announcers tried to keep the crowd at bay, but were running out of one liners and free give aways. The pack proved to be a harmless lunch, an electronic void station and one autographed baseball. The baseball brought in by the undercover agent? or had he made the switch already? It was anyone's guess at this juncture. A Mcguffin in an Alfred Hitchcock film, a clever tactic to create a diversion, to take the audience's attention or eyes off the ball and lead them astray to an otherwise needless prop. It piqued the curiosity of everyone around. The fans trickled back into close proximity to verify the authenticity of the baseball and the signature. Who did it belong to? A priceless item up for auction ? 'finders keepers?' pondered several security guards. The object in question far too precious and valuable to turn into lost and found. Their lucky day. It might as well be a multi million dollar lottery ticket. The sentimental value of the coveted leather clad sphere much too important to let slip though their fingertips. The crowd began to claw at the unclaimed prize creating a near riot and mob scene in itself.

**

Deep in the bowels of the underground CMDF facility near Bethesda Naval Hospital almost diametrically opposed to the ball park, a few miles away in NW Washington, the heart rate of all present and attending staff increased. The crew of the Proteus had arrived at the critical juncture in the operation. Do or die. They were now playing for all the marbles. Dr Mancini and the rest of the crew peered at the grey and white marbled appearance of the 'swiss cheese'. The necrotic, irreparable heart muscle and tissues were clearly demarcated next to the vibrant vital pinkish red tissue interspersed throughout it.

"My God! I'd give the president less than 50%" stated the stunned heart specialist.

"Approval rating?" questioned Dr Gum, not realizing his exceedingly slim chance of even removing some of the damaged tissue…

"Chance of survival" stated Dr Mancini somberly yet clearly. "If I didn't see it with my own eyes, I wouldn't believe it." No amount of medical experience, operative time or foresight could have prepared him for this spectacular mess. A hodge podge, pudding and pie, nearly brought tears to his eyes. They'd be in there for hours, maybe weeks he estimated. 10-20 minutes, the time that remained, even pushing it, every nanosecond of overtime now counted. He decided to triage the target site, remove the most obvious tell tale signs of irreparable tissues. Implant the cardiac stem cells deeply into the hollowed out furrows. Then, like any other farmer out standing in his field drop to

his knees, look up to the heavens and pray to God, for rain, a miracle, any measure of good fortune to fall upon him and the crew. Anything to cause the precious stem cells, nurtured, coaxed into the astronomical numbers now pending placement, to take root, sprout, initiate the totipotent growth processes. It could lead to a slow and steady recovery and a complete replacement of the existing non functional mesh of cardiomyopathic heart muscle now unsalvagable. It was his only hope and route to salvation, his resurrection it seemed. A donor match deemed impossible.
An artificial heart implant too risky in his present condition. They were his 'last best chance'!

"That bad huh?" asked Pam still amused by the amazing array of colors. To her it all looked so edible. Over indulgence and late night snacks the contributing factors that led to the present precarious predicament they all found themselves in.

"Have you found the target?" asked the CMDF commander anxiously. All the years of blood, sweat and tears, if only for this moment. Definitely worth the wait. All the decades of scientific inquiry, advances in medical science, the miniaturization methods, the cardiac stem cell discovery and mass cloning techniques seemed to converge on this pivotal moment in American history. If only to save a life it would have all been worth it. To save the president's life, inconceivable chilling, incalculable….

"It's huge" replied Dr Mancini, still in awe at the extent of the damage. "Beggin' your pardon, but president Taylor's created a monster inside his myocardium, uh heart muscle!"

"Can you repair it?"

"I dunno." He took a long deep breath, no better off from this angle or perspective as his heart picked up the pace pounding in his chest. "But we're sure gonna give it a try. It may take some time."

"Time, the one precious commodity we have the least of, we seem to squander the most…" insisted the commander as if losing hope. The odds heavily stacked against them.

"Life is all about timing. The unreachable becomes reachable. The unavailable becomes available. Have patience, it's all about timing!"

(Stacey Carter, cancer survivor). Pam hurried into the laser room and grabbed the life saver. Lethal in the wrong hands. A fine line between the two.

"The CO2's a workhorse."

"There's plenty of pastureland for grazin'. I'll set her down beside the barn door" quipped Sparks. He'd paid attention to the sermon on the mount by Dr Mancini and the others. He gently eased the Proteus to the large obstruction near the pulmonary trunk, the cavernous opening he'd estimated, presumably their best chance of escape. "Plenty of breathing room" he stated facetiously, no pun intended. In the face of insurmountable odds and grave danger, he had no time to think, merely react on gut instinct throughout his lengthy career as a nuclear submarine captain. Life and death decisions, each second now conceivably their last. By the grace of God they'd complete the mission and get out by the skin of their teeth. It was all uncharted territory from here on in. Dr Mancini visualized the rows of furrows along the folds of the semilunar valves. He used the membranous interventricular septum, the thick solid immovable mass, as his guide. The prominent pillar holding the whole house of cards together. If he incised too deeply the walls of the atria and ventricles could collapse or lead to a fatal 'hole' in the heart mixing the oxygen rich red blood with the blue colored consumed liquid.

"We can access the damaged heart muscle from here" he said as he pointed dead ahead. "A time to plant and a time to pluck up what is planted. (Ecclesiastes 3:1-8 KJV) I'm not a religious man but…" he looked up at the heavens. If ever he needed a prayer answered it was now. No time to wait for a message, they made their way to the hatch.

9: Rocket to Russia?

> 'Every gun that is made, every warship launched, every rocket fired, signifies in the final sense a theft from those who hunger, and are not fed, those who are cold and not clothed.'
>
> - Dwight D. Eisenhower, 5 star general of the army and the 34th president of the United States

The fans grew downright restless, a mob riot hung in the balance. Even the pitcher became impatient. He eyed the large pile of balls, and selected a few to wind up over home plate. The fans couldn't be contained forever. The show must go on with or without president Taylor.

The first lady concurred. They couldn't leave everyone in the dark. She decided to break the coveted code of silence.

"I think we better call, give them the head's up." The touchy subject demanded tactful diplomacy. The defense staff reluctantly patched her through. She cut to the chase and apologized; the annual physical by the team of physicians, was running a little late, behind schedule.

"Yes, I know he loves to plant his feet firmly on The mound and wing it from time to time. But he's still under 'observation', I'm sorry." Her firm yet subtle reply eased the reporters, press and stunned radio announcers.

"Now a word from our sponsor" they stated as they went off the air to discuss a few theories of their own. "What's come up? You know he's never missed a National's season opener" they declared as if it were written into the constitution, like a sacred vow or commandment, 'Thou shalt go to to the ole ball game!' or 'Thou shalt play ball!'

"The president as you know has been under a lot of stress." Wasn't everyone? with the state of the economy, the recession in full swing, the war on terror knocking on their back door, the nerve. He had an urge to give her a piece of his mind but refrained; it'd likely lead them to go off the air for good! Better to side with valor and better judgment and suck it up. Take one for the Gipper they agreed.

"Something's happened to him hasn't it?" pried the persistent straight from the hip shooter and radio talk show host.

"I can assure you" without giving away the farm, spilling the beans or putting her foot in her mouth, "....he's doing fine. He's simply under close observation." For lack of a better technical explanation and opening a whole new kettle of fish, neither she nor the VP knew the extent of the president's problem. In good hands under the guidance of the crew, she laid the issue to rest.

"Close observation?" repeated the relentless radio host. It sounded like either a poor choice of words or deliberate political psychobabble meant to bamboozle not only him but every fan in the ball park, should he decide to release the report.

"Closer than you can ever imagine" said the VP of

the United States softly thinking he was off the air and out of ear shot. It sparked a flurry of questions from the anxious announcer's. Fearing an ill fated physical, coupled with the terrorist threats, they suspected the White House staff may all be aboard Air Force 1 already, safely whisked from Washington, now under imminent threat of attack. The broadcaster broke down in a moment's lapse of sanity? sanilocity?

"It's part of the terrorist scare isn't it? You've slipped him onto Air force One. Why you're all aboard having a blast, cocktails and caviar chit chat, likely on his way to Cancun or the Caymans. While we're here …grounded…" and about to bear the brunt of the…...blast. He'd crossed a fine line between professional journalism and pushing a few of the first lady's buttons.

"Listen to yourself. Get a grip. We'll keep you posted" she said trying to restore the peace and trust like a small town sheriff in the wild wild west.

"Sorry, must be the sugar buzz from my soft drink" stated the reporter trying to extract the foot from his mouth and offer a rational reason for his out burst.

"I'm sure he wanted to be there like every other red blooded American ticket holder. Go Nationals" encouraged the first lady. The bitter pill no less palatable. The producer had to pull the program out of the fire back into the frying pan, expecting a grilling and bleacher full of boos from the loyal fans.

"Thanks ma'am."

The announcer had his work cut out for him as he cleared the air and dispelled any rumors circulating through the stands and went straight to a comical commercial.

"Play Ball!" hollered the umpire. He'd grown tired of waiting. It felt like an overtime inning in the 7th game of a World's Series. A deafening roar radiated around the capacity crowd as a small child approached the mound to sing the national anthem. The pitcher handed her the microphone. The child prodigy from a local church choir group struck the first few notes that resonated with the crowd. The audio system punched out the precious acoustics.

"…the bombs bursting in air…."

Inside the White House all hell broke loose. A series of intercepted messages and intelligence updates tipped off the secret service and staff to an imminent attack on the capitol. The first lady, VP, chiefs of staff, distinguished department of defense men were hustled into the bunker beneath the White House.

"Hurry, this way Mrs Taylor." Her immediate concern, the condition of her husband.

"The word is, all chatter indicates an imminent strike on the capitol."

"My God; is Air Force One…?" The plane still at Andrews AFB outside the perimeter of a small dirty bomb blast simulated to strike the heart of the city. All contingency plans were in place to allow a quick massive evacuation of all government staff and their families. The rest of the survivors, fleeing in a mass exodus, resulting from a hypothetical radio active ring soon to radiate from ground zero, were on their own. Several fallout shelters sat unoccupied. There was no warning. Not moment's notice was lost linking the capitol with the alternate command center aboard the presidential plane, and the 'doomsday' plane, a mirror of all ground based networks in the event of just a scenario. Rehearsed over and over redundantly in the drill, like an endodontist unable to locate and plug a painful 'flare up', the secret service and staff sprung into action.

"On its way" he said rushing her down a narrow corridor. Crouching down, and covering their heads from falling debris in an impending earth shattering blast likely to occur at any second.

The E-4 Boeing 'Nightwatch', the advanced air born command post was whisked out of the danger zone. Capable of launching all ground nuclear forces, primarily the nuclear submarines carrying the bulk of the deterrent strike capability, from the secure facility. In the event of such a scenario, the aircraft code named,'Looking Glass', shielded against EMP – an 'electromagnetic pulse', a debilitating electronic surge through sophisticated electronic channels and networks essentially frying the system and incapacitating communication's networks. All commercial flights were instantly pushed forward. The tarmac entrenched in aircraft enroute to any destination out of the capitol STAT!

**

"However far I may roam, there's no place like home" said the passenger near the center aisle midway in the aircraft. He savored the sweet elixir, good to the last drop.

"Let me take that" offered the friendly face inside the Dreamliner destined for the nation's capitol. A sudden diversion caused the pilots and several passengers severe grief and heart ache. The flight crew had to avert the congested compressed air corridor suddenly littered with aircraft. Unable to determine if they were landing or taking off, Sam, with superhuman speed snatched the drink from his tray and grabbed the stunned stewardess before she could grab his head set or took a cart wheel and potentially deadly tumble down the aisle; possibly upending the beverage cart.

The pilots were requested to divert to adjacent states and international airports immediately. In the most massive precautionary measure and movement of air traffic since 9-11, the ATC controllers tried desperately to rearrange the grid lock over the capitol and bring the blips down safely ASAP.

Eager fans were glued to their television sets throughout the local pubs, bars, hotels, vacancy rates literally nil due to the busy business and conference schedule this time of year. Anxious to toss the first pitch, the small child was escorted from the mound at center field. The pitcher rolled the ball in the palm of his hand. The accelerometer inside, piqued, primed, waiting a surge of information to set the sinister sequence of events in motion. Neither biased, nor aware of the outside world, the delicate sensors simply sorted through the barrage of information bombarding it from all three axes. Roll, pitch, yaw, X, Y, Z…the end. The omnidirectional device directly linked to the detonator of the nuclear device placed some where inside the stadium.

A homeless bum outside the stadium discovered a baseball in a dumpster and a shiny suitcase. He reached down to grab the dirty weather beaten leather sphere.

"Must be my lucky day. My luck must be changin'?" he declared his toothless grimy grin, spread across his face as the pitcher spread his palm around the baseball to unleash a rocket across home plate. He wound up whipping the ball over his shoulder like tossing salt for good luck, then snapped his wrist. The bullet blasted from his hand, straight as an arrow at the crouched back catcher's mitt. Before it covered more than a few meters from the mound, the adept accelerometer sent the fatal signal to a silver brief case left near the 'suggestion box'. Out of sight but not out of mind. The cold calculated premeditated device, left there, as if the president or any other staff would ever honor his request. The madman satisfied with his clever highly orchestrated scheme. A brilliant flash consumed the darkness and much of the air over Washington and the Navy yards alongside the Potomac near the ball park. The immediate hiatus then sucked up the molecules in the concerted chain reaction and spit them out over ground zero. The searing shock wave melted everything in the immediate area. Steel ships crumpled under the intense heat wave. Airliners instantly incinerated caught in the flight path of the atoms dispersed like an aerosol over DC. A massive shock wave reverberated through the planes near the perimeter or outer reaches of the blast zone. The pilots fought feverishly, having lost all control guidance and electronic systems in the aftermath of the electro-magnetic pulse from the small kton nuclear blast.

The E-4 absorbed the atoms and molecules hurled at it. The resilient skin and sub structure of the aircraft especially designed to withstand such a shock wave, remained relatively stable and airworthy. All systems were go as it replaced the immediate irreparable damage to knocked out, vaporized ground stations.

Many television viewers glued to their screens, their drinks raised to their lips, their speech stopped mid sentence, the countless citizens leisurely walking their dogs along the mall, or in a green belt near the White House, were instantly incinerated, many left little more than a wisp of a shadow indelibly etched on a surface.

Sam sensed the shock wave; he recognized the wretched beam at blinding speed as it enveloped the aircraft. The pilots were powerless to intervene as the Dreamliner dropped like a dead duck from the sky. Their only hope to keep the nose up, and ditch somewhere along the Potomac now aflame. The former American naval might, the naval yards had taken a direct hit, nestled along the banks of the Potomac near the National's Park. Neither an accident or random attack. The terrorists knew where, when and how to cause considerable damage. Their prime target, the president, presumably consumed in the inferno. Unaware of his whereabouts, somewhere a few miles from the epicenter in NW DC. The gruesome route, a grim reminder of the menacing awesome power of splitting the atom, now lay in utter ruin. Rubble and debris littered the streets. Former famous landmarks and monuments unrecognizable in the immediate vicinity. Museums reduced to rubble. Models of the Monitor and Merrimack now mere molten metal, likely the fate of many an ironclad vessel, or sunk to the bottom of the river after a proud period of service. The scene, right out of an apocalyptic Armageddon type thriller. Something straight from a US target practice range or deadly tsunami. The nuclear blast had flattened everything within a few mile radius from the detonation point. The naval yards, officer's quarters' and mess, were obliterated.

The pilots aboard the Dreamliner negotiated the fiery surface. Flat, hard, flames rising like the devil's lair itself, yet miraculously they managed to bring her home on a wing and a prayer. The petrified passengers thanked Almighty God for their deliverance. Neither out of the woods, which looked like the devil's cauldron that consumed Chernobyl, nor peril yet. The boiling bubbling stew, a scene from Hades brought the passengers and crew to their feet. They resourcefully punched the exits and swiftly evacuated the plane. Out of the frying pan, and into the fire…many feared no escape. Some preferred to stay aboard and take their chances, go down with the plane rather than face the searing heat. Yet the river was probably their best means or way out of the immeasurable mangled mess. Former frames of fast frigates and missile cruisers littered the shore and percolating waterway. Several survivors crawled to the tip of the wing. The life rafts deployed, they made their way through the surreal nightmarish landscape. Hell on earth many described the gruesome hellish inferno. Sam paddled toward the far river bank relatively certain of what had happened. He had to lighten the load of flotsam and jetsom and jettison, his jittery petrified passengers. Drop them off, emergency fall out shelters scattered throughout the city still sound, safe havens out of the immediate impact of the radiation, scorching heat and smoke. His first thoughts, the condition of the president and the Whitehouse staff. Why was he forced to come back to this wretched inferno in the first place? Were they witnessing the end of the world? A fatal first or even second strike in retaliation to a Russian or foreign invader? With no means or channels of communication open to him, the only option to confirm his suspicion was to make his ways through the dilapidated war zone to Bethesda Naval Hospital.

The blast ripped through the ER. The path of carnage completely ravaged the rest of the facility. Glass shards were blown about, as each pane was pushed out by the tremendous force of the shock wave. The OR staff was bowled over like balsa wood. Lying next to toppled iron lungs, ventilators, heart monitors, IV drips, patient charts and papers lay strewn about, some still smoldering in the sooty residue that covered the floor of the institute. Patients in beds, troops just home from the battle front to relive the horror all over again. Shell shocked and disoriented they crawled through the rubble unable to distinguish the alien landscape.

Critical care units were annihilated. The shock wave surged through the surgical wards. Several oxygen and anesthetic gas reservoirs exploded. The nurses and attending worked feverishly to extract any survivors and those still breathing faintly, clinging to the last breath of life, from the inferno. Several staff had just awoken, knocked out cold from the blast. They peered about the place, speechless, still in a state of shock. A few patients slowly picked up the pieces of their shattered lives and rummaged through the rubble for any discernible signs of the living in the land of the dead.

The reporters scrambled to cover their heads from the sky literally falling down upon them. They were standing patiently inside the hangar waiting for the news helicopter when the worst case scenario they'd often elaborated upon in one of their own broadcasts, broad sided them. The hangars collapsed or were instantly incinerated. The thick grey sooty snowflakes sunk to the floor of the former aviation facility, obliterated in a heart beat. The news caster salvaged a Sony hand held TV camera cowering over it like a precious little baby.

"Get us up in the air STAT!" they insisted still unclear of what had just happened. The thought of a nuclear strike or brief case nuke detonation hadn't sunk in, all merely idle chatter, conjecture for a compelling news story at this juncture.

"Sir?" questioned the puzzled pilot. His simulated combat training painted a clear picture as he fiddled with the war bird, under repair at the back of the charred hangar. He peered across the sooty console, then knew what had happened. The airworthiness or the aircraft in question, he demanded to know the source of the spectacular albeit shocking 'first strike'.

"EMP knocked out the entire console" he stated to the reporter, relaying the most reasonable explanation for the horrific explosion. A retaliatory strike likely in progress provided the White House and Pentagon were not gone. He had to desperately restore a communication link with the outside world somehow. "We might be able to wheel her out onto the tarmac, but that's all she…" wrote? The writing was on the wall. The second strike now a matter of minutes away he estimated. He had to assess the damage. See if there was flight capability and sufficient firepower to launch even a small resistance force. Where and from whence it rained down thunder and lightning still a complete mystery to most. It struck without a warning other than accelerated chatter and one very ominous FOX report. The news reporter suddenly grasped the gravity of the situation and thanked God he was still very much alive.

Through hundreds of feet of solid rock below and around the perimeter of the blast zone, which now lent credence to the theory that the Chesapeake and Potomac around Washington were once struck by a sizeable meteor 35 million years ago. It created the permanent 'depression' or crater like formation similar to those found on the surface of Mars. The circular souvenir now clearly demarcated. Not of extra terrestrial origin but by a self inflicted wound from a man made monster. Inundated, partially mitigated by the multiple strata of prehistoric layers, the EMP had done considerable damage to the CMDF. They felt the earth shake under their feet. The atomic clock had stopped. 30 minutes into the procedure, now closer to midnight, a formidable warning of an impending nuclear holocaust and complete annihilation of our species.

The computer consoles and screens went blank. Much of the sensitive dense sophisticated circuitry was fried in an instant. All communication links with the outside world were instantly severed. The elevator shaft stood silent, immobile, rattled from the resounding shock wave and sudden rush of soot and debris that fell from the surface. The lights flickered in the eerie surreal kaleidoscope light show as the emergency diesel generators slowly kicked in. Most monitors, ipods and cell phones malfunctioned. The electric underground now reserved to a few vital functions like forced air and emergency light, water and power. The staff wondered what happened.

"It's DC sir."

"I don't care if it's AC or DC!" fumed the commander. "Just get us back online!" he crawled out from under the inoperable terminal then laboriously pushed himself up onto his knees then a prostrate position as if learning to walk all over again. Humbled, brought to his knees by the earth shattering experience.

"That's Washington DC sir."

"What is it?"

"It's gone sir!" stated the stunned staffer dropping the dead buzzing receiver.

The CMDF commander realized how small he and his mighty military really was as he peered over to the patient. As if expecting an immediate response and order to initiate a retaliatory strike. He couldn't yet ascertain if the commander in chief was dead or alive. He just kept on hoping and praying for a sign. Anything, a peep from the president.

10: Heart of the Matter

'Destiny is not a matter of chance, it's a matter of choice. It is not a thing to be waited for, but a thing to be achieved.'

- William Jennings Bryan, 19th c. politician, lawyer, military colonel

A few of the computer screens and monitors came back on line. It was not the pretty picture they envisioned as they arrived and reported for duty earlier that day at the first rays of the dawn's early light. Everything outside lay in utter ruin.

The blast had decimated DC.

The catastrophic power failure left everyone focused on the president. Had he survived the brunt of the blast? Had the heart lung machine continued to push the vital life sustaining liquid through his brain and vital organs? Or was his mind reduced to mush, rendered a mental and physical vegetable? And what fate awaited the crew? Were they still in the swing of things as the fateful pendulum struck another glancing blow upon the mission. Perhaps ill fated from the get go? They'd placed the chances of a full recovery by the president at 50/50. The feeble attempt to patch his heart with unproven albeit potentially priceless cardiac stem cells sheer conjecture.

The Proteus was riveted by a shock wave of immense proportions. Sparks had taken evasive action wondering whether the surgical staff had inadvertently restarted president Taylor's heart prematurely. All signs indicated a tsunami like tidal wave emanating from inside the circulatory system somewhere. The indeterminate force slammed the submersible hard. The GPS, gyros, and all navigational systems and onboard computer circuitry failed. It flung them about inside the dense mesh work of chordae tendinae like a fly slapped by a fly swatter at the worst possible moment. Pam was knocked out cold draped over the laser about to disembark. Luckily still tethered, it teetered precariously, her finger near the trigger poised to apply pressure. Dr Gum had hit his head against the front plexiglass view port and too lay unconscious on the cold steel floor. Spared the front row seat to witness the smashing entry into the wall of the heart. The sub, now immersed in the cardiac muscle like the survivors of the SS Minnow, stranded on some God forsaken distant shore. Neither three hours of saving grace period, nor a coast guard chopper or a return trip aboard the Love Boat could save them now it seemed. The pilot was pinned into the upper compartment attempting to avert a head on collision and likely sever a set of strings supporting a heart valve. Yet the ball kept bouncing, the 'bucky balls' had come undone from the pouches, and bounced about further mixing totipotent mixtures of cardiac stem cells like tossed salad or a lucky Lotto Power ball lottery. Their luck seemed to have run out. The sands of time were slowly running out. Not the deserted tropical isle any of the crew would wash up on someday as they might've envisioned. They now faced the cold harsh foreboding land scape face to face and on their own. They had to salvage whatever flotsam and jetsom that they could, vital to the completion of the mission, and flee, fast. Complete the groundwork; patch the space and head for the nearest exit. Split second decisions now meant life or death not only for the president but themselves. Dr Gum awoke with a splitting headache that radiated from the back of his cracked and bleeding cranium. The bouncing bucky balls grabbed his bleary eyed attention.

"The stem cells!"

He raced to reach them. The floor and ship's artificial horizon askew, the gyros malfunctioning, he slid and lost his balance and hit the deck. The anatomical heart charts lay strewn about. It appeared as if a brutal struggle had taken place aboard the vessel. Mutiny or cunning sea pirate capture attempt, all he knew was it was time to get out. The macrophages would soon gain wind of their pesky presence and initiate a welcoming committee. Not the warm wide armed variety awaiting them should they ever return to the outside world like astronauts at their home coming; but a cold ruthless, merciless slow death as if at the hands of terrorists intent on torturing them until a ransom was paid. Clotting would soon commence with or without the aid of the heart specialist who slowly propped himself to his feet. He braced himself on the sharply angled counter wondering what hit them. Dr Gum sequestered his wild imagination to focus on the task at hand.

"Couldn't hit the bright side of a barn, huh?" He complimented the pilot's precise placement of the Proteus, pinned to his perch. No reply left them shivering in their boots. One of their worst fears realized. The only one who knew his way around these parts passed out, possibly dead. The heating system had also conked out, not uncomfortable, slightly below body and room temperature. The crash had likely also killed the controls and 'engine'.

"I don't know what hit us, some sort of shock wave?" suggested Dr Mancini, mortified by the possibility they'd restarted the president's heart without them and prior to their departure. Had the clock run out? Sparks finally came around. The pilot peered at the dark fleshy folds dangling in front of his face outside the plastic bubble. Miraculously still intact, the panorama left him spellbound. Embedded in the heart muscle, only adding to and compounding the problem plaguing the president. He couldn't self destruct now nor escape. No time to think, they had to get out STAT!

"Must've been some sort of electromagnetic pulse" he reasoned suggesting the only rational explanation for the sub's catastrophic system's failure. Which meant only one thing. They, the CMDF and conceivably the entire outside world was under attack. He didn't want to alarm the rest of the crew needlessly. They had their hands full as it was. A million miles from home. First and foremost, the team had to fix the failing heart before it was too late. Roger reached down to remove the tangled mess of electromechanical parts on his lap.

"From a nuclear blast?" wondered Dr Gum groggy, but a firm grasp of the gravity of the situation. "I can only imagine what happened up top?" All eyes looked up, relatively speaking, and imagined what might've occurred. Ironically safely sheltered, buffered from the blast, down below in no man's land. The one man they had to save, had saved them. They owed him more than a mountain of debt and gratitude. They owed him their lives as his fate now rested entirely on theirs.

The surgical staff breathed a sigh of relief, their worst fears abated as they scoped the surgical apparatus. The resilient die hard Maquet heart lung machine hadn't missed a beat or regular roller coaster ride of the relentless rollers and pumping action. The emergency power supply had kicked in and shifted into high gear giving president Taylor a fighting chance. The staff cheered, and encouraged one another, brushing the dust and debris from each other's shoulders and grey lab coats. One more strike, against them but the game was still on. Late in the bottom of the ninth inning, the base of the heart loaded with the bravest souls, about to attempt to hit a home run and bring 'em back alive!

What happened?" wondered Pam. "Were we hit by a tidal wave, surf's up?" she asked. Her wetsuit slightly torn, a trickle of blood ran down her forearm. Not deep or seriously enough to warrant her to abandon the mission or finicky gun fight. The delicate task of obliterating the deleterious plaque still rested with her. The weight of the entire world suddenly upon her, squeezing, adding to the inscrutiable pain that radiated from her separated shoulder. She screamed in agony. Not of victory but imminent defeat. Dr Gum fumbled with a syringe, the damned device that landed them here in this hellish nightmare in the first place, and shoved it into her shoulder. The lidocaine numbed her shoulder and clavicle and sent a shot of adrenaline surging though her veins. Just the jump start she needed to finish the job. Dr Gum helped her to her feet. Together they untangled the delicate lasing instrument and prepared for final departure. The vessel had served them well. All's well that end's well? Oh well? Worse for the wear and solidly embedded in the heart muscle, they gathered their few belongings donned their scuba masks and gear and departed. Roger had released himself in the nick of time to join the three amigos. The four skin divers now on their own in the strange alien undersea world for the first and likely last time.

“Change in flight plans” declared Dr Mancini as he beelined for the main target site. What a mess he mused. “The other side must want him badly, dead or alive” he lamented unsure of his present state. Was he still breathing? Alive? The small steady current reassured him the heart lung machine must still be working. A good sign from the outside world. Had they weathered the storm? Survived a first strike? A nuclear holocaust unleashed? He placed their survivability on an even playing field with that of the president. They may be better off here inside the warm wet under sea world like the inviting womb, the prenatal wonder of child birth. Neither the world nor time he’d want to bring a newborn into.

“Like they say ‘he inherited half his father’s friends and all his enemies’,” (George Bush quote) stated Dr Gum realizing the extent of the wall to wall damage facing them. They looked back over their shoulder at the ship. Such a colossal concept, such a tiny ‘toy’ submarine, like the one’s most of them had played with in their youth. No time to reminisce.

"She's a goner. The ship's lost all navigational control. We're on our own from here on in" fretted Roger, they'd have to make it up on the fly as they went along now. The game plan squarely on the pitcher or quarterback. The playing field so much larger than life. The reality of the situation required a quick remedy and concerted effort. Pam was to blast a few deep incisions into the loose flabby folds of grey fleshy 'moldy cheese'.

"We came here to finish a mission, and by golly that's what we're gonna do!" The renown surgeon felt so small and insignificant about to ask Pam for a scalpel as she examined the laser for leaks or ruptured lines.

"Superficial scratches. I don't know if it still works?"

"My balls are still intact" stated Dr Gum eyeing the entire two large spheres he held in his hands. Cautious to check for cuts, tears detrimental to the delivery of a full soccer ball full of stem cells. Secondly not to let them drift out of his hands, downstream, and jeopardize any chance of a successful completion of the mission.

"Glad to hear that" chuckled Pam. The tiny bubbles emanated from her scuba mask using up precious compressed air. It temporarily disoriented her, as she aimed the laser scope erratically in the air.

"Come on people" stated Dr Mancini pointing to his deep sea diver wrist watch. He raised both hands fully extended. 10 digits signified the obvious. "We've got ten minutes to implant the cardiac stem cells." The outburst consumed the precious ounces of oxygen that remained. As I said I'm not a religious man but I think this is a good time to pray he mused.

"Oh God get us outta here" stated Pam suddenly overcome by the sheer magnitude of their dilemma. She let er rip like quick draw McGraw. The laser plowed through the pillowy dead folds of flesh billowing from the upper reaches of the chordae. They fell like feathery light gossamer wings revealing the bright ruby red under lying healthy heart muscle. Scattered about, then soon sucked out through gaping valve like refuse from the mild albeit noticeable current. Dr Mancini conducted like an aging relic of the Boston Pops, directing her to separate the wheat from the chaff at key strategic points. They'd never clip the entire crop of cardiac muscle that had simply ceased to function. 'Reap what one sowed'. It seemed so bizarre, an unbelievable feeling enveloped the crew. The fate of the free world rested in their hands. Such indescribable power, yet at the same time, so small and insignificant. It was a humbling experience. Comparable to standing on the moon and looking back at the earth in the vast emptiness of the universe. Unable to gauge the elapsed time, Dr Mancini had severely miscalculated, assuming they had at least five minutes, sufficient to flee from the surreal scene.

**

Sam hurried and paddled the small dinghy filled with a handful of patriots across the Potomac much like Washington might have felt crossing the Delaware. Neither the first move in the surprise sneak attack nor likely the last. No one could fathom from where the next bombs might come. The rockets red glare burning brightly on the horizon as crews onboard the badly battered naval vessels salvaged what little that remained of their former illustrious fleet. A few gun batteries, and even a couple deadly Sea Sparrow missile rocket launchers remained intact. Intent on sleuthing out the notorious unknown nemesis in a heart beat. An adversarial outpost or enemy target impossible to determine at this place or point in time. The survivors struggled to reach the shore then clawed their way from the rubber life raft. Crawling, clamoring up the shore of the parched putrid panorama of the once pristine picturesque Potomac. The passengers were shaken and stirred. Their escape from the burning fuselage now as dicey as the final descent into the unfolding drama. Sam turned back and slowly watched the wreckage sink below the surface of the burning oily waters of the river. He had to move forward, to the heart of the matter. The question burning in his brain, 'where was the president? Was he still alive? The only answer lay somewhere deep below the rubble he assumed. A considerable distance from ground zero. Bethesda may not have survived the blast, but the chances of fewer casualties bode the CMDF well, buried deep beneath the NW outskirts of DC near Chevy Chase and Friendship Heights. Nothing appeared remotely friendly nor of significant height in the desolate diorama forever changed in a flash, flattened like a compressed pancake. Sam crawled to what might've been a walkway or former fashionable thoroughfare at street level. It was difficult to gauge any reference point or landmark in the garish gruesome erratic terrain. The flesh fell from those few souls that had survived the initial impact of the blast near outside ground zero. He presumed somewhere to the south side of Washington. The White House, Mall, capitol and state buildings were no more he assumed scouring the thick smoke, debris and rubble to the north. The naval hospital still worlds away due north west. It was like entering a bizarre surreal video game. The object, to navigate the alien landscape and rescue the heroine, the damsel in distress. Damn it! he fumed; how did things ever get so miserably out of hand? He decided to go it alone in the decrepit bombed out backyard he once called his home. The grim backdrop continued to burn mercilessly making emergency access by the first responders practically impossible. A few robots had penetrated ground zero to determine the cause of the blast. The tiny motorized eyes and ears rolled overt the rubble that only moments earlier had stood proudly as a pillar of American society and accomplishment, National Park Stadium. The obliterated bleachers were all that remained. Indelibly etched in the wrecked remains, shadows, of happy, thriving souls only seconds ago, instantly incinerated in a flash. Sam sought a way out of the macabre panorama. He spotted a few burnt out charcoal shells of what appeared to be checkered cabs, completely blackened by the impact of the blast. Most of the roadway, possibly Pennsylvania Avenue remained under feet of rubble, twisted and contorted shredded steel and aluminum frames. There was no sign of life. Countless cars and buses were flattened or unrecognizable. Buildings obliterated, erased in the aftermath of the eye opening event in the wink of an eye.

Miraculously a yellow cab surfaced from the smog, smoke and mirror reflection in the wretched waterway. The driver must've crossed the bridge in the nick of time just out of harm's way before it too collapsed and sunk into the Potomac.

"Bethesda, on the double!" demanded Sam out of the blue. The disoriented pale faced driver, his turban singed a shade of dark grey, stopped and opened the door. Glad to see another human being and more signs of life, he eagerly took the fare. He brushed the dusty dashboard, and pulled the lever on the fare box in a trance. The windshield had been blown out, glass shards were scattered across the front seat. He didn't seem to see nor care in his shell shocked state. All that mattered was to accept the stranger and take him to wherever he wanted to go. Amidst the turmoil the cabby wondered where the wayward wanderer had originated. He didn't mean ethnically or country of origin on the face of the earth either.

"Where did you come from?"

Sam was lost in space, in deep thought, dazed and confused, both at the sight of the cab and the causes of the catastrophe. A spine chilling revelation raced through his brain.

"The other side…." He answered hesitantly in disbelief. He paused for a considerable length of time mulling the millions of thoughts darting through his subconscious. "Might be winning the 'inner space race'," he rationalized. The meaningless statement might as well have been Greek. The petrified driver looked vaguely like Peter Sellers in 'The Party', his face plastered with soot or shoe polish to portray the East Indian guest at the respectable dinner party. This was neither the time or place to bring up pleasantries of a palatable wine or dessert. Their dry parched palates sought any drop of moisture not contaminated by the radioactive fallout likely rampant at epidemic proportions in the immediate vicinity. The NEST teams had not yet arrived to ascertain the extent or composition of the radioactive cloud hovering over the capitol region. Their immediate concern to initiate the carefully choreographed simulated disaster recovery scenarios over and over. In situ and vivo everything looked much worse than it was. The years of painstaking planning for just such a hideous horrific event would hopefully pay off. The intense, in depth disaster plans prepared for every contingency option conceivable. They took careful aim to arrive at ground zero while dealing with the heart of the matter; how to save the survivors of the unimaginable carnage and indescribable destruction that had befallen Washington.

Sam realized the other side must've either gotten hold of the miniaturization methods or planned to throw a little more than a monkey wrench into the mix to impede and thwart the delicate operation. Yet, one thing he couldn't quite put his finger on was, how they'd found out where the president was unless… He licked his forefinger then raised it into the air as if to check the wind direction or to flag down a cabby. A redundant gesture thought the taxi driver, impatiently waiting for his fare. He brushed the glass from the seat making his rusty rent a wreck more presentable.

A military chopper appeared miraculously out of the blue from amidst the thick smog. Like a guardian angel watching over them from above, its bright floodlights sought out the two survivors. Either his subatomic signature had tipped them off discernibly difficult to distinguish from all the other particulate matter floating around the region, or just a lucky hit and miss, a shot in the dark. He knew not as the noisy bird of prey descended, kicking up quite a wake. A couple armed soldiers dashed form the door which instantly opened as they touched down.

"Need a lift sir?" asked the trooper. Had he picked Sam out from the crowd? "We've come under heavy fire." They maintained their position around the cab, a vantage point, if only to a virtual unknown target.

"Friendlies?" asked Sam glad to see the soldiers reassuring him that the capitol nor country hadn't capitulated completely following a crushing blow.

"Nobody seems to know where it's coming from sir." Inspite of the confusion, the soldiers seemed to know who he was, and presumably where he'd come from. And decidedly where he was going. Certainly not on his way to the forum or quorum. The number of survivors so far and few between at this stage he was lucky he wasn't the solo or lead in this passionate portrayal, drama in real life. He could only lead them to where he thought the president might be, safely tucked away in the underground lair. Lucky to have missed the fire works. That is if he hadn't tossed the first pitch at the home opener. His heart leapt and missed a few beats as he brooded over the bewildering turn of events. The soldiers led him and the cabby into the aircraft out of the immediate danger zone. Pockets of gunfire had erupted from the general direction of downstream along the Potomac. Resilient rebels determined to fend for their city, confused, shell shocked yet proudly defending the flag until the last man fell.

11: Beat of a Different Drum

> 'If a man does not keep pace with his companions, perhaps it is because he hears a different drummer. Let him step to the music he hears however measured or far away.'
>
> - from 'Walden' by Henry David Thoreau, American author

The gunfire originated from one of the vessels in the small flotilla maneuvering through the burning debris and rubble littered midstream. A steady stream of bullets and small mortar fire flooded the sky. The fierce gunmen, possibly minutemen determined not to go down without a fight.

What unfolded next was indescribable. Sam caught a glimpse of the flag waving from the bow of one of the boats. Tattered and torn, the Bolshevik or Russian hammer and sickle or variant thereof. Like a virtual video game aimed at prepping the next generation of warriors, he found it difficult to distinguish between fantasy and reality. An awful thought struck him in a flash. Had the other side discovered the secret of 'miniaturization'? Not only a crew and small submersible, but an entire fleet? He tried to perish and suppress the thought. But the startling reality of a Russian retaliation in their own backyard was right under their noses. The only logical explanation, a defector or GRU agent had cleverly slipped them into the country undetected, minimized, concealed in luggage, Samsonite to add insult to injury. Mocking him, the American secret weapon and the highly coveted technology. If his worst fears were realized, it meant the inner space race had entered a whole new era, a new chapter in counter terrorism and international espionage. A new type of cold war was likely to ensue.

"Those aren't friendlies! I know this sounds so far fetched…but…" he didn't know whether to spill the beans or not. He'd likely have his guts spilled all over the cabin if they sensed he might be an enemy agent himself or secret spy withholding important information, especially enemy combat plans. Torn, he decided to tell the whole ugly truth…

"The vessels were enlarged." The soldiers laughed, ridiculing his sound reasoning, a lapse of judgment on the battlefield. Shell shocked; he'd come to his senses once he received the medical attention he so desperately deserved now.

"Those missiles seem larger than life alright! You're still in shock." The soldier tried to calm the citizen unaware of his true identity. "Come on, we've got to go now! Which way you goin'?…" he wanted to say Billie but hadn't even asked his name yet.

"To Bethesda Naval Hospital. How hard was it hit?"

"Pretty hard. Bethesda's in ruins…" he replied somberly. As the Pavehawk crept slowly into the smoggy air, a few former landmarks became more obvious. The soldier pointed out across the river as the pilot took her hurriedly out of harm's way. Not wanting to get caught in the crossfire below, he veered over what once was Washington proper. The vibrant political nucleus lay torn apart like a predatory attack by a cancer, metastasizing, spreading its deadly path of destruction to every adjacent cell. Too bad it hadn't sought out selectively the location of the terrorist cell in time.

"The epicenter was in the naval yards over there. Uh.. the infield took the brunt of the blast. I just can't figure for the life of me how the ships survived the blast?" The bewildered the soldier removed his hardhat and sat on it to protect his privates. He scratched his sweaty sooty forehead in a futile attempt to figure out the rest of the topography that looked like a tsunami or hurricaine had swept the city like Katrina.

"That's what I'm tryin' to tell ya" fumed the flustered CMDF agent. "They're not ours! They're Russian ships!" he declared defiantly. The soldiers shared a hearty laugh.

"What? You're shell shocked" as the soldier and part time paramedic checked Sam's forehead.

He reached out and felt the skin yet could not ascertain if the rise in temperature was from the immediate heat of the inferno of coming from within the delirious DC resident. “You’re making no sense at all!”

Sam pointed to the vessel coming upstream.

“Up the Potomac!” he snapped.

“Impossible!” denied the soldier with a mind to take them both as detainees. The East Indian seated silently opposite him shrugged his shoulders oblivious to anything Sam said. He was merely along for the ride. The first yet possibly his last time aboard a military helicopter he sensed.

“Anything’s possible!” Sam sat in utter shock, stupefied by the rapid Russian assault in the midst of the mayhem. The events must be related he mused. “They must’ve found a way to shrink their forces for a significantly longer period of time.”

“Brings a whole new meaning to ‘may the force be with you’ don’t it?!” humored the soldier as the helicopter slowly veered off and headed in the opposite direction. The pilot had orders to peruse the Bethesda blast site. Signs of survivors and attempt to gain access to the CMDF entrance if at all possible.

"You can say that again! Our forces took the knock out punch from the nuke." How the Russian raid had survived the shock waves, still a mystery to them all. "A small 6 kton nuke from the size of the collateral damage" he estimated. "Then they simply sauntered up the lazy river. They planned to take the capitol by hook or crook." A ludicrous, far fetched plan thought the soldiers focusing on more urgent matters immediately at hand.

"Pirates on the Potomac, who knew?" wondered the weary war vet. The military maven mulled the possibility of the ship's insertion into the Potomac somewhere downstream beyond the blast zone. Nothing could've withstood the impact of the explosion near the docks, a stone's throw from the baseball field. A deadly distraction to divert the attention away from a full scale assault?

Down below a drama was beginning to unfold. Like a recreation of the battle of the old ironsides. Only this time, the tango entailed two much more modernized vessels. Heavily armed with surface to surface missiles, overkill in the close confrontation, literally hand to hand combat as the ships approached like the ancient armadas, practically ramming one another as they prepared to board each other's vessels.

"Get down!"

Bombs burst all around them in the air. Caught in the fierce cross fire, flack flew in the thick smoky response of both sides. The copper crew took swift evasive action to get out of the immediate 'no fly zone' immersed in shrapnel and flying debris flung all over the once friendly skies. The Pave-hawk responded by unleashing it's own ATS, air to surface propellants in a futile attempt to repel the Russian flotilla.

Sam's head began to spin. He felt a strange sensation, side effects from the electromagnetic pulse? His pym's particles repositioned, realigned? dispersed, scattered from their quantum orbital paths? His superpowers of little use in this, the final confrontation anyway. Like a fly about to be swatted out of the air, he knew they had to get out of there STAT! Hurry to their objective, as the helicopter hovered over what was left of the multistoried medical facility. Windows were blown out, Sliding glass doors, reduced to wrinkled metal frames some crumpled like contorted coat hangers. The parking lot was reduced to a used car junk scrap heap. Impossible to uncover an entrance the Pavehawk helicopter touched down in an empty depression, a former parking space? Sam scrambled across the smoldering debris, racing to the remnants of the renown medical treatment center. The show of bodies still shuffling about was a welcome sign of life in the land of the dead. Bewildered, scarred, bleeding from every orifice, sooty from the debris like a front line MASH unit; the patients, waiting room attendees and staff were in a state of confusion. The victims were quickly triaged then whisked into the bowels of the building, somewhat removed from the perimeter which had taken the brunt of the shock wave. The helicopter, EMP proofed prior to the mission, managed to maintain radio contact with the rest of DC and a few residents inside the battered building. Some systems and secondary power supplies, such as diesel generators, slowly kicked in. It kept the crucial ICU and cardiac patients heart's beating in tune to a different steady drum beat. Sam stepped up the pace if he were to reach the CMDF in time. At this juncture he feared he'd find nothing but a collapsed crushed shell of what remained of the revolutionary facility that rivaled Bethesda in terms of it's mystical healing properties. The entrance to the long deep elevator shaft that reached toward the center of the earth was nowhere in sight. Toppled cars, ambulances and special care vehicles topped the list of wrecks. Their hollowed out shells a reminder of the force of the atom and mother nature or that of a deadly devastating hurricaine. He sifted through the staff, their pale parched forlorn faces forced a weak smile by the mysterious visitor. Like a ray of hope amongst a group of untouchables, they hadn't given up or lost hope yet. There was still a sign of life amidst the hellish inferno. A straw to clutch, and that civilization as we know it hadn't completely capitulated. They asked him to offer his services to tend to the wounded, the weary and the sick. He humbly denied, insisting his indigenous inherited possibly God given superhuman talents be better utilized elsewhere. He declined and continued to cut a path through the facility to where he recalled the secret entrance once lay.

Evidence of the earth shattering explosion was everywhere. Recently dressed patients were copiously applied with new salves and bandages. The most critical cases were hurriedly wheeled into newly formed ICU's in lieu of the crushed equipment and spirits standing outside a series of former life saving series of wards. Their grim demeanors said it all. What had happened? Why? where did the deadly blast originate? A terrorist attack? was world war III upon us? Neither long on answers or opinions at this point, Sam raced through the rubble. He knew his time was short. He had to find a way to get into the facility. Cut off from the rest of the world. The fate of the free world now hinged upon the clear and present danger of the president's passing. A second strike imminent, likely already ordered in lieu of his absence. To prevent a further catastrophe on a global scale he hurried to find a way 'in'. The outsider had always lived on the fringe. Neither fully human nor superhuman. The cards had dealt him a deadly blow much like the blast. Subjected to a phenomenal experimental military procedure, Sam had practically been atomized in a bizarre atomic test. His molecules or pym's particles, as they'd been dubbed, were instantly rearranged. He'd miraculously survived the instantaneous transformation. The highly unlikely survival coupled with an even greater garish capability to shape shift and reduce his size almost at will boggled the minds of the top military brass. It caused an immediate brash response to enlist the oddity, the freak of nature, and most promising miniaturized 'WMD' or tactical response mechanism in the ongoing war against terrorism. The weird weapon, or micro miniaturization method, literally shrinking at will was a valuable adjunct to the CMDF. They hoped they'd no longer need to place entire crews into jeopardy.

Submersibles or other military paraphernalia, the puzzling quantum physical phenomena neither controlled nor understood. A by product of the blast? His molecules scattered across the universe, drawing matter from a black hole upon itself? Theories and speculation tossed around like a hot potatoe, as much as the circus freak that he had become. At times, when the intensity of the interrogations became too much to bear, he'd simply 'disappear' from sight for a while, from the entire human species it seemed. Yet no place on earth was remote enough or out of reach. How and why they had found him in the tropical paradise in ironically 'Micronesia' of all places, a mystery to him. A dead ringer giveaway.? He only knew he was summoned for another top secret mission, to assist the crew of the Proteus. Priority One. It usually meant a matter of life and death he'd learned from past missions. And to prevent him from defecting to the other side, they'd rewarded him not only financially but with considerable leeway to conduct his research fully funded by the NIH, CMDF and other NSA departments to discover the cause and conceivable 'replicability', if such a word existed; to recreate the ideal conditions to 'atomize' then recreate or 'remolecularize' another human being. They feared the secret may be soon lost forever, along with the last traces of the 'incredible shrinking man'. The rarity, perhaps from birth? Destined to denature, part of his inherent nature? The presence of the metagene, found only in a few extremely rare cases, the gene that predetermined the possibility of a full transformation to a superhero. Why fate had bestowed the bewildering blessing or curse upon him, still unknown. He knew he had been given a gift. Yet with great power came an equally compelling compliance to use it for good. Not for evil purposes. He followed in the footsteps of so many former super heroes, to the tune of their own drum, a highly unique hyper accelerated beat at times. Far beyond the comprehension or capabilities of mere mortals. How long the super powers would remain was anyone's guess. As quickly as it had happened it could all be taken away in the wink of an eye.

There it was again, that strange sensation, surging thorough his body. It made him feel queasy uneasy. It had no noticeable side effects, at least not yet. A product of the atomic blast? To return him to what he once was, a mere mortal? An ordinary human being? Functioning on a biological clock in tune to the rest of humanity? Driven by the clock and internal innate mechanisms bound to run down in a preprogrammed genetic dance. The repairs and replications of vital genes all numbered like the hairs on our heads? No high tech rocket science there. For we are all appointed once to die. He knew not where and when, simply that he had evaded the grip of the grim reaper once again. He had to make the most of whatever God given talent and time had left to find the president. It was why he was saved in the plane crash and from the blast he figured. A chance for him to shine and give back. Where mere mortals dared to tread he raced ahead boldly. Sam soon reached the boundary of the bombarded building, a no man's land. It must be here somewhere? Neither fearing death or debilitating radiation burns which he must've suffered upon his initial arrival in DC, he danced about darting across the debris like a Mexican jumping bean or grasshopper on crack or speed. He stopped to scour the scattered sections and singed structural components of the hospital one more time. The smoldering pieces of the jigsaw puzzle just didn't seem to fit. It was then and there, when the night was darkest before the dawn, that he spotted a small ray, a glimmer of hope depending upon one's perspective, like the two last port authority survivors stranded, buried several stories below the rubble near ground zero on 9-11. He zeroed in on the source of the strange light. A flashlight? a security guard must've dropped it in the ensuing events? A parking lot or car light left on, the batteries about to die? He clawed his way through the rubble, tossing flotsam and jetsom aside. As he removed the layers of strata, the array of light shone ever brighter from an unknown source. It reached up into the heavens as if to signify 'we are here', we are all still here and very much alive! He inched toward the edge of the precipice and teetered over the edge. He braced himself and peered into the abyss. The gaping rectangular hole clear evidence of the manmade marvel. The CMDF headquarters and center was indeed still very much intact and alive!

The soldiers had painstakingly followed him through the crowds of people perturbed by his erratic elusive behavior. Their sole mission to provide protection and support enroute to his target. He needed nor wanted either. The soldiers rushed toward the stationary target, relieved he'd stopped. His pace was wearing them out. They couldn't maintain it much longer weighted down by the full battle gear. The advantage of progress? Of being able to atomize oneself at will? It had certain advantages at airport check out lines. Reduce the size and weight of carry ons, usually on his person, slipped into his CMDF emblazoned polo shirt pocket. Anything in close proximity to him, much like that of a body caught in the clutches of a black hole, could be significantly reduced in size. He didn't ask why, merely went along with the flow.

It all seemed to lead to the edge of the crevice, or the known universe for all that mattered? leading to the center of the earth as far as the soldiers were concerned. They kicked some of the larger pebbles over the edge. A significant drop for one man, let alone for mankind. They had to figure a way to lower themselves into the manmade illuminated aperture. The elusive landmark, the obvious unmistakable target in question.

**

Diametrically opposed near downtown DC, Marine One had touched down in a small clearing near the what remained of the capitol buildings. The gutted garish grim landscape, bore no resemblance to its former stately appearance and grandeur. The hollowed out hallowed halls, the dome destroyed, the east and west wings, now mere figments of imagination for future restoration experts and fond memories of the past. The splendid structures that lined the promenade frequented by as many as 24 million people a year, sat silently smoldering in the after math of the ghastly monumental societal altering event. A few million had perished in the wink of an eye, without cause, rhyme or reason, other than to prove a point perhaps? that such monstrous mayhem was possible? the might of the atom never in question or doubt. The deadly delivery devices despised, determinedly and decidedly to disappear from the face of the earth by all delegates. A unanimous universal decision to eliminate the WMD's entirely from the face of the earth came too little too late. The long term lingering effects from the fallout would be felt for hundreds conceivably thousands of years. The scarred landscape and buildings replaceable. The irreparable detrimental damage done to the remaining citizen's inherent molecular makeup now the main concern. The inconceivable carnage of the capitol paled in comparison to the reconstitution of their genetic make up. The deadly ionizing radiation, likely to leave scars for generations to come. The residents of Chernobyl could testify to that. The hideous humor of 'free xrays' still haunted them. The 'red forest' a grim reminder of the radioactive cloud that clearly swept across the countryside for hundreds of miles. Estimates of the extent of this tragedy were forthcoming. The turbulent windswept eddies carried the contaminated debris aloft, some into the outer reaches of the atmosphere, along with a pollen dust and natural debris. Dancing about in the sooty stale ionized air, perhaps a swift somber deliberation for some, slow lingering painful death for others. The familiar sounds of traffic, trolleys, tourists failed to resonate on the survivor's eardrums. The sound of laughter, of children playing in the park, had ceased. Instead a somber eerie silence, marked by the intermittent cry of a dog who'd lost his master in the macabre inferno. The sound of air traffic ceased, other than the EMS and first responder swiftly entering no man's land. Only the intermittent sound of gunfire remained, in the surreal ravaged zone near ground zero, like a territory torn apart from war and constant strife, the citizens stifled and silence, destined to serve the successors who followed in the footsteps of the fallen. The troops swarmed the perimeter of the virtual parliament buildings as the secret service hustled the first lady, staff and senators out of the bomb shelter. They met halfway near the steps of the Whitehouse. Beelining toward the birds of prey, they prayed and shed a few tears at the sight of the utter devastation all around them. The war vets and national guard whisked them aboard the helicopter out of harm's way, what ever that meant at this juncture. The damage had been done. All eyes and focus of attention eagerly now focused and waited upon a swift stern reply by the president. A display of determined resolve and show of considerable force to dissuade a second strike and to mitigate any impending international military engagement.

"What about my husband?" wondered the awe struck woman. She could not process nor fathom the full extent of what she saw.

"Bethesda was hit hard. We don't know much damage the CMDF sustained. We're still trying to restore communications." They tread where eagles only dared. A few singed corpses unhinged even the helicopter pilot. He hadn't seen anything on this scale other than the simulated flight training through just such a scenario. He anxiously waited for the last of the politicians to board. An endangered species in this neck of the woods he feared, "Come on Mrs Taylor, we have to hurry!" They couldn't miss their ride, a one way ticket on Air Force one and an immediate pass out of the parched wasteland.

12: Take a Stab at It

'Actions speak louder than words.'
- Shakespeare,

'Well done is better than well said.'
- Benjamin Franklin, American

Safe inside the hermetically sealed helicopter. The electronics systems onboard the billion dollar bird buffered from any EMP or enemy fire. The pilots bore down through the dense irradiated fog, giving off an eerie garish red glow. Several squadrons of F22's, F35 JSF, veered into formation to create a formidable offensive line that soared across the Potomac, a distinguishable point amidst the emaciated earth. The precious pristine channel now carried the dead downstream, grim reminders of former battles of the past. Nothing on this scale, so fast or furious crossed their minds. Still jarred from the jolt, a harsh reality and worst wakeup call imaginable in Washington's history.

"My God! How could we have missed it?" wondered the bewildered woman who may soon face the biggest challenge of her life. To step into the president's shoes. Replace the respected world leader and take over his heart wrenching responsibility. A daunting task that no one cared to entertain at the moment. Yet a decision had to be made soon.

"He didn't miss by much!" declared the dignitary as he perused the barren wasteland lucky to get out by the skin of his sooty teeth.

Would the president ultimately step up to the plate and make an appearance no matter how fashionably late? Or had he already succumbed to the shenanigans, the stress his ailing heart had been subjected to and taken his place amongst the illustrious leaders of the past. Perhaps at the worst conceivable moment in the country's history.

The warning lights in the helicopter suddenly lit up like a Christmas tree. Bells and whistles clang like a church wedding or referee's response. The pilots instantly deployed chaff and decoy in a last ditch effort

"My God, those are NOT friendlies!" came the blood curdling scream from the copilot.

"I don't know how they did it, but the Russkies are here" stated the startled seasoned vet scanning the cockpit console. He took every step and evasive maneuver to avoid a direct hit. "The Russkies, or whoever they are, brought more than carry on with them!" as the scanners detected the sizeable flotilla directly below them. The counter measures barely kept them air born let alone afloat. A direct hit likely to upend them and toss them mid ships or down into the flaming depths of Davy Jones' locker room.

"We've got illegal aliens up the wazoo and now they're firing at us too?" Where, how, and when they'd entered the country causing such a calamity still unclear to all aboard. Certainly why amidst the questions posed by their befuddled expressions. "Just get us the hell outta here" barked the belligerent commander in chief's spouse, ready to let 'er rip and assume the coveted leadership role. The billion dollar aerodynamic marvel weathered the barrage of incoming shrapnel, missiles and unidentified flying debris formidably. The feisty featherless bird of prey evaded the ensuing second wave, surviving the EMP. It flew them out of harm's way by erratic evasive gyrations and gut wrenching twists and turns. The very superstructure moaned and groaned from the excessive G forces. The pilots' paw prints now indelibly etched in the joy stick by his unrelenting grip and determination not to take a nose dive into enemy hands. Several more situational awareness sensors piped in the particularly annoying status report. As if the computerized defenses had kicked into high gear. The entire defense department was taken to DefCon 2. Neither the time nor the place, the lag time since the actual attack warranted a Def Con 1 response. He tapped the gauges and wished he could turn back the hands of time to a few moments prior to the sneak attack. To negotiate a peaceful settlement or settle the score any where but upon American soil.

"Ma'am, the president has to call off an imminent counter strike!" screamed the copilot, assisting the commander like riding side saddle upon a bucking bronco or ornery steer. 8 seconds had come and gone. They'd managed to keep the bird afloat yet could not control the bearings or omni directional tail spin. Her tail feathers clipped in the process, spinning perilously out of control.

The passengers grabbed onto any piece of the powerful frame holding the glue of the fuselage together to avoid being flung form an open door, damaged by errant gunfire.

"You mean he has to be present?" snapped the stunned first lady about to be thrown out of the helicopter. Her legs dangled over the edge of the outer hatch as she hung on for her life.

"Yes, I'm afraid so" declared the joint chief of staff as he reached out to grab her outstretched hand. The presidency and spousal support hung in the balance as both senior staff were about to be sucked from the aircraft. As they reeled the resilient woman, who'd reached menopause, yet not once pausing or slowing down one iota, into the aircraft and stated,

"Well I wouldn't want him to miss the fire works," defiantly. They dragged her onto a sumpfy leather couch, worse for the wear, and buckled her up. Front row seats and much more than any of the stunned spectators bargained for. She set her hands into her lap, and prayed. Nothing they'd ever planned for or conceivably envisioned in their wildest dreams, now right in front of their faces. She wanted to shut her eyes, wishing he were here. But what of it? He had his own slough of problems to deal with. He hadn't married a quitter. The hard headed debutante, determined housewife and deliberator of the family finances, who sought to wade the waters, now in it up to her eyeballs and find a way out of this mess, and bring some sense of order out of the sensitive situation. Mismanaged the media warnings, severely under estimated the determination and drive of the demented madmen responsible for this heinous act of cowardice.

The staff aboard Air Force One had immediately gone to Def Con One awaiting word of the leader of the 'free' world. Neither free, oft taken for granted, peace came at a heavy price, incalculable casualties and cost on this occasion. The president's appearance was warranted to sway a determined and deliberate blow to knock the wind out of the sails of the sizeable marine assault. The assailants in the air or on the ground as of yet undetermined as the intelligence reports rushed into the onboard computers. Billions of bytes of data digested to select the safest route to intercept Marine One after it left Andrews AFB, then to haul their asses out of the inferno. They were all lucky to be very much alive at this juncture in time still shaking in their seats. They peered out over the barren parched wasteland and wished they had eradicated the WMD's weeks, even years ago when they brought the issue to the bargaining table mulling over them like mere board game widgets.

Marine One made its way across the Potomac out of enemy fire. As valiantly as Washington had traversed the Delaware. Their focus on a rapid response by the naval forces, that had banded together in a haphazard albeit heated resistance. The JSF 35 squadrons surged out of the clouds like white lightning sending bolts of fire and brimstone in the form of SAM missiles and an assortment of potent paraphernalia raining down upon the enemy crews and gunmen. The runways were quickly cleared as waves of fighters soared skyward. Flooding the former friendly skies with a welcoming committee the hostile takeover teams wouldn't soon forget. The sneak attack and veritable vanquish of valiant troops soon turned to a stalemate, like former fierce water born batteries, their six shooters and guns a blazin' from the surface of the water. They were gradually winning the war. The tide was slowly turning in favor of the feisty formations coming together like powerful magnets. The small pockets of resistance began to repel and contain thc cunning pirates of the Potomac.

Time, the one precious commodity the president had so aggressively clung on to yet could neither recoup or reclaim, seemed to be running out. The grains of sand had slowly slipped away. The hour glass nearing its final fatal few crystal fragments. His absence would be dearly missed mulled the staff of the CMD. Their long forlorn faces could not imagine the impending plight of the fearless crew now desperately fighting to flee the presidents ticker. A ticker tape or victory parade now only a distant remote possibility. They had lost all communication with the vessel following the fatal blow DC had been dealt below the belt. The intermittent signal signified a catastrophic system failure, perhaps even a lethal nuclear leak into the patient's bloodstream. The weak pulse like a fading transponder sending its last breath from a tropical isle, the fate of the craft now in jeopardy, like a castaway. Coupled with the fact that it resonated from the same stationary position meant only one thing. The vessel had lost its navigational system guidance, control and likely crashed into the cardiac muscle, permanently lodged in president Taylor's heart. Not the heart warming reality they wanted to hear and likely relive over and over again soon. And what of the crew? Had they been killed? Or trapped inside the Proteus to face a fate far worse than death. The swift deterrent forces would soon find them as their approached the end of their miniaturized life span. They'd soon begin to grow to enormous proportions not only endangering themselves, but the president and the entire immune system. Sensing the foreign invaders for the first time, a rapid response from natural killer T and B cells, the formidable host defenses neither hospitable nor friendly. They'd soon be caught, chewed mercilessly like a child eating its food at a Christmas or Turkey dinner, giving thanks; then mercilessly swallowed possibly alive by the macrophages, and predators percolating from strategic outposts in the lymphatic system. Soon racing to the scene, to initiate a swift aggressive assault to thwart the invasion of the president's private personal inner space. All was lost they feared. Their chances of survival slim to nil. They'd all but lost hope in the ill fated mission. The unprecedented unexpected events had thrown them a curve ball. The fatal third strike. There was no time to ponder possible courses of action nor mull over a million coulda shoulda, wouldas now. They needed to act fast!

Through the smoke, a dark silhouette emerged. As the sooty life form drew nearer, the stunned staff soon realized who it was. The sweaty dark facial features, so familiar. The tiny unassuming frame, equally discernible. He had entered the

CMDF headquarters on many an occasion before. The silent guardian angel, like a sentinel in the midst of all the mayhem, had arrived, likely hovering over them waiting until the last moment to grab them from the clutches of the grim reaper and the jaws of death. With a slight limp, yet brisk pace the superhero entered the badly damaged facility. Tarnished, its reputation and perfect record of wins and no casualties, in jeopardy, Sam smiled and approached the commander ready to report for duty.

"Well, well, aren't you a sight for sore eyes? Sam," then extended his hand in a firm filthy fingered hand shake. Both brothers in arms embraced in a teary eyed encounter.

"Glad to be back sir." The unassuming, even frail character soon got up to speed and the status of the project in as few words as possible. They lost no in briefing him in only the basics and bare essentials then led him to the miniaturization chamber, hopefully still functional. They placed their chances at 50/50 to bring them back alive even if Sam found them in the nick of time.

"Most of the facility is inoperable. The

president's heart is still tickin'...takes quite a lickin'. He's still on life support" he stated uttering a prayer softly to himself. "It's touch and go!" He looked at his watch and ushered SAM into the OR. "There's no time left!"

The superhero, his marvelously deceptive metagene and incredible shrinking ability now seemed like the only hope of reaching the damaged heart tissue and initiate a patchwork quick fix let alone find the crew. It was worth a shot. A long shot as the OR nurse prepared another syringe for vaccination and insertion purposes. Only likely a one way ticket she figured. She hated to be the harbinger of death like Jack Kavorkian. Each time she'd inserted the syringe into the forearm of a patient lately, she felt as if she'd deliberated a death sentence for, at times multiple victims, men, women yet fortunately no children as of yet.

"Looks like your luggage arrived" stated the commander facetiously, luckily not rerouted amidst the rest of the airline fiasco facing the capitol and not aware of the origin of the initial blast. Yet one average sized briefcase, determined to be the cause of the chaos that rendered the capitulation of DC.

About to embark like a doctor without borders, the ill equipped superhero, other than a back pack, scuba gear and a prayer, summoned the strength to initiate the 'atomizing' phenomena. Sam positioned himself near the hypodermic on a stainless steel tray. Without further ado he focused intently to carry out the fantastic shape shifting transformation.

"All is not lost, you know what to do!" as he nodded before the knowledgeable OR scrub nurse.

"Aye, aye" she stated in with sooty smile.

The superhero activated the 'pym's particles by depressing a switch on his super utility belt lens. The vets wished him well while the new recruits watched in amazement as the incredible shrinking process began. He quickly shrank to the size of a youthful paperboy, about to bring good news to the crew. Then a small child, a baby, then rapidly to a Ken sized Barbie doll quickly reducing to a miniature fighter found in a table top recreation in famous battles. He stood next to the towering hypodermic. The graduated marks now like rungs on a ladder. He hopped onto the bottom rung then rapidly ascended to top like a high diver aboard his lofty parapet or smaller than a fly in the ointment. Sam peered over at the president's extended arm. It reached out like a vast desert.

"Must be his pitching arm" came the tiny squeak from the tiny figure standing on the rim of the syringe.

A burst of laughter emanated through the room that nearly bowled him over off his lofty perch. Sam weebled but wouldn't fall into the salty drink.

"Sorry!" whispered the nurse finally grasping the ramifications of radical reduction, neither a simple procedure. She wondered what might have happened to the crew and sub from the catastrophic albeit mitigate EMP they had to endure likely the cause of their stationary present circumstances.

Sam leapt off the plastic perch in a spectacular swan dive arc receiving nothing less than perfect 10s from the judges. He waddled around the circular swimming pool awaiting his fate, now squarely on the shoulders of the skilled OR nurse.

"This won't hurt a bit" implying pain to the heavily sedated patient or Sam in the center of a raging torrent in a few seconds. He smiled awaiting his fate. The scrub nurse carefully inserted the plunger. The sudden darkness enveloped Sam, like a tropical thunder cloud encompassing most of a mini isle in Micronesia. Somewhere he wanted to be, anywhere but here!

The nurse approached the president. By careful palpation she counted the number of ribs from his clavicle then located the landmark. She jabbed the syringe as if administering a lidocaine bolus directly into the president's heart to otherwise normally revive a patient. Sam was instantly tumbled like a tiny life raft in the midst of a raging hurricaine or tsunami or an unscripted underwater synchronized swimming routine. End over end, he hoped the dizzying dilemma would end quickly. He began to have his doubts. His worst fear realized. What if she jabbed him into the middle of the interatrial septum, the dense muscular wall separating the left and right sides of the heart. Or worse, way off the mark into the lungs. He'd soon succumb to gale force winds albeit muted during the heart lung machine perfusion. Or worse embedded in a mass metastasized myocardium, at the mercy of an organized macrophage attack, definitely behind the front. Likely consumed quickly in a concerted counter measure. His mind was too small to amuse a million ifs racing through it. If only he'd missed the flight…

"May the force be with you!" urged the general, the CMDF commanders and host of innocent bystanders. He, president Taylor and the rest of the crew were in God's hands now. No one could even venture a guess about how they'd get out. From a fresh perspective from inside the patient's heart chamber, a large stainless steel projectile pierced the pericardium, then penetrated the inner lining of the blood filled atrium. The end of the hypodermic needle entered the left heart chamber.

Pam noticed a large projectile, like a large Satan Russian missile, a dud, delivered near the sub. It had luckily missed the target.

"Are they shooting us…er at the president?" opted Pam, putting two and two together. She presumed the shock waves were attributed to a terrific earthshaking tremor on the capitol. As she swum to investigate, indeed it was a large cylinder. A bullet? Had an assassin breached the tight security and attempted to end the operation and the president's life? Penetrating the pulmonary trunk narrowly missing the Proteus. She reached a point below the shiny metal mass and discovered it was hollow. A hypodermic? venturing a guess. Ready to repel the assassin, she raised the laser defiantly. Shoot first, ask questions later? Sam grabbed the rim of the angled aperture to gain his bearings. He peered up from the edge out onto the alien landscape. A curvaceous creature of similar cloth slowly lowered her weapon. Obviously a woman noted Sam, slowly recognizing the familiar face. A smile, then chuckles from inside both masks. A barrage of tiny bubbles erupted as Sam crawled from under cover of the hypodermic tip. They embraced briefly then released each other in the presence of the rest of the rattled crew.

"All it takes is one navy seal" surmised Pam, happy to see at least one reinforcement. Her elevated heart rate, both at seeing the swarty superhero and drastically increasing their odds. Sam scoped out the garish scene.

"What's a nice girl like you doing in a place like this?" he questioned, which made no sense to her by the surge of bubbles. The formidable task at hand still not a cake walk, or walk in the park. The reddish inflamed tissue reminiscent of the red forest encircling Chernobyl comparable to the vegetation around the capitol he mused. He noticed the sub trapped, embedded in the heart wall. A few moments now separated all of them from life or death. A deterrent force would soon be dispensed from within the countless blood vessels and body's lymphatic forming tissues.

"It's a bloody mess" as he assessed the massive walls, like two colossal slices of bread buttered with raspberry or strawberry jam. "A sticky wicket on both sides.." Neither the time nor place to have a quiet peaceful breakfast. The floodgates would open at any time unleashing a bone crushing torrent of blood or blood borne macrophages set to feast on the tiny palatable hors d'oeuvres.

Dr Mancini was elated to see an assistant and an extra set of hands. His renown surgical skills of little use he found on this magnified playing field.

"Am I glad to see you! I owe you one!" declared the disgruntled heart specialist.

"We have to hurry, we only have a few minutes."

"And the sub?" questioned Pam pointing the laser to the vessel that had served them so well.

"The antibodies will have a hay day. Hopefully no room left for dessert…er us!"

Dr Gum grabbed the bag full of bucky balls as if going to a soccer practice. Pam, presumably a soccer mom, carefully followed to catch any balls that may fall from his sack. Dr Mancini led them to the most obvious scene of catastrophic damage. Pam had sliced several deep furrows with the CO2 laser, forming sizeable rows in which to insert and plant the massive 'seed pods'. The bucky balls containing the priceless totipotent cardia stem cells were pushed into the fleshy billowing folds of tissue.

"Take your best shot!" Before Pam could take aim, the balls had worked their way out of the furrows, the planting had come undone, about to be dragged off by the current. Any hope of a golden harvest gone. Sam resourcefully reached into his satchel and produced a handful of ugly slimy gyrating creatures.

"Sea cukes, they release a sticky substance when provoked and an anti clotting factor." The man and scientist for all seasons and disaster scenes, applied a generous serving of the sea cucumbers onto the pumpkin sized medicinal packets. They attached themselves like Velcro or double sided sticky tape. Dr Gum reinserted the remedy into the rills. The crew stepped back and watched as Pam performed the last act in desperation. Like laser welding or placing the final sutures to close the wound. The laser, on its last legs, sputtered and fizzled out. The soccer balls ceded and began to release their seeds of hope as the final weld was closed. They'd have to wait and see if they'd reap the rewards of their monumental efforts.

13. The Buck Stops Here!

'I never gave anyone hell. I always told the truth and they thought it was hell.'

- Harry Truman, 33rd American president, businessman, farmer (chapter title also his quote)

Time had run out. The pesky search parties of natural killer cells, macrophages and a whole host of body defense mechanisms sprung into action. The golden hour, pass go card had bode them well. The crew became a growing menace shortly upon the expiry time as they lingered around the president's private parts. Now considered loiterers languishing in the cavernous vault they had no time to think. Their immediate concern to get out while they still could. Growing to the size of similar clots and plaque, they'd soon plug up the constricted blood vessels, easy prey and target practice for the B and T lymphocytes bearing down upon them. Sam sensed they didn't have time to reach the intended targets, still miles, nowhere near the fingertip. The tiny survivors might as well be swimming in an open sea miles from anywhere., the nuclear sub, their only transponder, other than Pam's malfunctioning ankle bracelet. Sam hurriedly hauled a number of deceptively light nanotubules from his back pack. They looked like tent poles. Neither the time nor place to set up base camp, or stay for a while. They had to get out NOW! The tiny nanobots began to reassemble and rearrange themselves into an organized network of small pentagons and hexagons, in a type of mechano set reconstruction. The quickly unfurling framework, similar to a giant bucky ball. The C60 carbon nanotubular Buckminsterfullerene formed right before their eyes. The delicate slender skeletal structure was swiftly covered in a thin sheer membrane like a tiny time release capsule. Each diver now safely inside their own hermetically sealed environment. Pam and Dr Gum shared the same sphere, as Sam had run out of extra 'life boats', two to tango, tossed about like a giant transparent water ball or water walker.

"Walking on water are we?" asked Dr Gum dumbfounded. The event more miraculous than the rest of the unbelievable adventure. The membranes seemed to selectively exclude and osmose only the oxygen from the fluid and soon dispelled the rest like a hatch aboard the Proteus.

"Like two peas in a pod" chuckled Pam. As the water receded and levels dropped in the bubbles, Pam dared to remove her facemask. She was amazed to find, indeed, the sphere was saturated in a rich reservoir of breathable oxygen. The only drawback, a fluid to buffer them from the impending rapids as they were about to leave the slower pooled bloody slough in the heart. If the president were to be forseeably revived in the near or immediate future, the experience may toss and rattle them about like a rattlesnake's rattler. The balls soon slipped into a stronger suction and swirling eddies out of the tricuspid valve up into another larger cavernous space.

"Times up" stated the CMDF commander sadly. All eyes were glued to the atomic clock. There was no signal from the crew or sign of progress from the ill fated mission. The Proteus' persistent bleep embedded in the heart wall like a nuclear pace-maker, continued to emanate a small steady virtual heart beat.

"They must've fled" assumed the general. The statisticians and analysts assessing all possible options.

"But where to?"

The crew had little choice in the matter, as if by fate to follow the bouncing ball in the lead position. The hermetically sealed enclosures continued to upend and swirl about tossing the inhabitants to and fro like patients in the padded walls of a room in a psych ward. The strange sensation, mitigated by the fact that the near invisible nano film was a strong impervious semi permeable membrane. Sam was left without an enclosure., soon to face the ravages of the resistance forces welling up in the president's body. A terrible feeling in the pit of his stomach caused him to crouch and keel over. He sensed he must have suffered some sort of insidious side effect following and in close proximity to the nuclear blast. He didn't know what to make of it, and followed his heart and the last of the balls being swept away by the formidable current.

Pam pressed the palms of her hands against the thin almost sheer veil powerless to intervene, now merely tossed about like flotsam and jetsom in the vast sea of blood.

"Merrily, merrily, merrily, life is but a dream" she began to sing mesmerized wondering where they were heading and where it would all end? The persistent pumping action of the miraculous work horse, the Maquet 20 Heart lung machine continued to draw deoxygenated blood into itself. Via the plastic tubes leading from the presidents SVC and IVC into the ports of entry, the blue blood was swirled about by the relentless action of the rollers that spun in a never ending circle midway form the attachment points and the machine per se. The buckyballs like all the other effluent matter or vacuous empty red blood cells depleted of their life sustaining mixture, were sucked into the out going tubes.

The surgical staff watched and waited patiently. A perceptive surgeon retraced the lines leading from the president's heart to the Maquet 20. He imagined himself in their shoes, facing a similar plight. What would he do? Where would he swim to?

"If I had to flee…." he mused at length. "I'd head for the heart lung machine." He turned to the perfusionist as he followed the intricate network of tubes and lines leading in and out of the machine. Through the oxygenator, the heater to ultimately bring the prostrate patient chilled to reduce basic metabolic rates, back to body temperature.

The perfusionist on a similar line of reasoning, hopefully the right track focused on the two lines leading toward the rollers spinning along pressing and squeezing the blood by sheer gravitational force unto itself.

"The grapes of wrath?!" stated Pam as she peered ahead into the distance. The tubing narrowed radically suddenly. Another clot? or constriction in the president's plaque plagued plumbing? It suddenly donned on the heart specialist seeing the same ominous picture from the lead ball, that they'd entered the starting gate or transfer point into the bypass system. It was anyone's guess what the inevitable outcome of the race would be. They braced themselves inside the balls expecting the worst. About to be crushed, like a select Napa valley vintage at harvest. The fine grapes pressed, squeezed into another enticing elixir that taken in moderate quantities might've prevented their departure in the first place. Everything in moderation they mused. The unimaginable images neither comprehensible or pleasant. The surface of the tubing quickly constricted as the full force of the rapidly spinning roller bore down on the plastic life line. It grew dark as the distant operating room light disappeared. The world was cast into utter darkness for a few nanoseconds. Not the bright light at the end of the tunnel they'd all heard or read about at the end of the line, their life lines. The pause proved to be unbearable as they awaited their fate. The bucky balls narrowly slipped through the cracks as they evaded the massive jaws of death, about to be filtered like filleted fish through the baleen strainer of a great whale. The balls emerged on the other side out of harm's way, a world away, yet not out of the woods by any means.

The perfusionist postulated and came up with an idea. Unproven, he approached the heart lung pump. An uneasy feeling in the pit of his stomach soon enveloped him. He had no time to think.

"It's a long shot, but here goes..." he stated as he reached for the plastic cap covering the reservoir of blood nestled between the series of pumps, that spelled certain death and oxygenator and heater certain to sizzle the small entities. The surgeon adeptly clamped off either side of the reservoir for a few seconds. Sheer terror filled the hearts of the bewildered surgical staff. Had he gone mad? cut off the patient's blood supply? What was he thinking? The perfusionist pushed a large operating light affixed to a magnifying lens over the reservoir to assist in his desperate search. He scoured the surface of the turbulent sea, like a coast guard SAR helicopter crew. Desperate to spot any SoS or sign of survivors. With no time to spare, the surgical staff about to push the two crazed men aside, he suddenly spotted four giant 'beach balls' for lack of a better description. He recognized them as the never used before nanotubular bucky balls in the event of just such an emergency.

"The buck stops here!" he declared. He reached across the operating table and hastily grabbed a rubber eye dropper and aimed at the small speck on the surface of the sea of blood aided by the optical lens. In one swift motion he swept the survivors onto the slick smooth transparent surface. The crew didn't know what hit them. An errant tidal wave? Proteus or Poseidon, likely to succumb to either death by misadventure at this juncture they mused.

The perfusionist placed the drop of blood onto a glass slide delicately next to the president then stepped back and prayed. The forms inside the bucky balls began to grow like small embryos inside a transparent pliable shell. The bodies began to take on a human adult form and soon breached the nanothin membrane and slipped to the floor as if expelled from the womb in a slimy watery birth. The stunned members of the crew coughed up a brackish surfactant, then peered about unable to fathom the transition. Flung from the deepest darkest crevices of president Taylor's heart, to the inner sanctum of the surgical suite, his secrets safe with them. The commander atop his lofty perch took a head count. Only four crew members of the ill fated expedition returned.

"Where's Sam?" snapped the stunned seasoned commander. He'd seen and heard it all in his day.

"MIA, missing in action" said Pam as she unzipped her tight suit a fraction and peered about, as if to greet them all in her birthday suit but refrained. It'd likely give a few senior staff a heart attack she figured, present company excluded. The all too familiar words, not the news he wanted to hear. He'd sent many a man into harm's way before in desperate attempts to extract his men form behind enemy lines. He hadn't expected this. Not from a super hero. More human than any of them could've surmised. Sam's selfless act of heroism would long be remembered, inevitably forever.

"Must've been a side affect of the aftershock of the EMP" stated Dr Gum taking a stab at the cause of the catastrophic system failure aboard the

Proteus before Sparks uttered a word. Foremost on his mind, the briefcase embedded in the wall of the heart muscle. The same nuclear device set off in national park Stadium? The president's ticker, still a ticking time bomb about to go off, literally?

The somber mood and silent reflection turned to one of equal compelling uncertainty.

"And the mission?" questioned the clever perfusionist.

"A success!" stated Dr Mancini jubilantly, catching his breath. Premature, presumptuous? "Implanted, we'll have to wait and see if they grow" he said nervously. The seeds of hope had been sown. With a lot of TLC, the first lady and family by his side, an attentive talented surgical staff, they were certain he'd weather any storm.

"MIA, myocardial infarction addressed" stated Pam. Sam's efforts neither unnoticed nor needlessly in vain. There was no sign of the super hero in the turbulent sea as the perfusionsit continued to scour the surface for a sign of Sam.

"Glad to hear that!" offered the general, appreciatively. "He'll be up and at 'em (atom?)

in no time" he concurred.

"Just in time for his presidential address" quipped the quick witted dentist and amateur appointed aquanaut.

The staff let off some pent up steam and emotion in a brief celebratory cheer following their tenacity and persistence. The surgeon placed his hand upon the shoulder of the perfusionist as if to say, 'you can be my wingman anytime.' The mission completed on a wing and a prayer. The casualty count limited on one lost soul, lurking somewhere presumably inside the president's heart.

The staff of the boisterous facility was suddenly bombarded by static and endless chatter, the broad cast the result of sudden restoration of a few communication channels, even if only emergency military frequencies.

"I'm afraid he'll have to address the nation STAT and without his teleprompter!" stated the commander urgently. Evens had escalated and were spiraling out of control from what he could surmise.

"Commander come in, this is Air Force One, over. We have a 'situation'!" The understatement of the century, the flight crew had inadvertently restored strategic links to the under ground lair. Perhaps in a last ditch effort to ascertain whether the commander in chief was still coherent, capable of offering a few conciliatory, kind words to the rest of the world gone mad.

"What the devil…who is this?" he barked. He demanded to know what game was being played and who had the balls and arrogance to call themselves AF 1 over the secure channels. They could neither confirm nor identify the source of the signal in the state of utter disarray of lifelines.

"This is mrs Taylor, I'd like to speak to my husband. This is an emergency. No, this is a state of National Emergency!" she responded precisely and deliberately. Level headed with all of her faculties intact inspite of flack and shrapnel flying all about AF1.

Uncertain of the authenticity of the caller, he had to play it safe.

"I'm sorry, he's…he's recovering" uncertain of the state of the president; awaiting a status report from the surgeons any second.

"He's alive?" asked the first lady, about to burst

into tears. She kept her cool iron clad composure. She'd withstood the shock wave, the heat, and was ready to face anything in hell's kitchen.

"Very much so" insisted the commander confirming the source of the transmission that originated from on board the bird of prey. He prayed and thanked the Almighty, that He'd seen fit to grant the USA another day, even if by the grace of God. That there was a world to return to, albeit at present unbeknownst to any of the trapped tired and mentally taxed staff.

"Good, then get him on the line or we won't have a free world to run."

"What do you mean?"

"We were hit pretty hard! A preemptive strike." She along with the majority of the defense chiefs of staff figured. She had to be sure and not jump the gun at a random act of terror. "Intelligence sources suggest a rogue Russian faction. A rebel arm of GRU, planted a small nuclear device in National Park." The epicenter clearly demarcated from the crater sized remnant inserted inside the preexisting prehistoric crater like shell from the

Chesapeake to DC and Maryland.

"An octopus' garden?" questioned the commander. "Ha, they've gained a foothold in the Russian capitol as well." The commander had either lost it or blown a 50 amp fuse. They knew not which. The rest of the blank pale faced staff did not understand the underlying meaning of the phrase. This was no time for charades, only second opinions to avert and all out world war.

The joint chiefs of staff puzzled by the phrase, unlike any other prearranged launch code to initiate a second strike. Their hair triggers hovering above a globe about to push the button and obliterate Moscow.

"We've been trying to restore all communication channels with Moscow. For all we know, the Kremlin might've been targeted as well."

The military montage of DC was a surreal scene out of a table topping tournament, at this point no clear winner in the obscured charred topography. A stalemate imminent in the stale putrid irradiated skies. Several squadrons of fighter jets were scrambled from neighboring airfields to repel the Russian armada slightly outnumbered by the seemingly irreparable damage done to the naval ship yards.

"The president must be awoken immediately" snapped the joint chiefs of staff. To initiate 'Snap Count', the final sequence of events likely leading to the end of the world as we know it or to make sense of this colossal mess.

"The world needs to know my husband is still very much alive and well and in complete control of his faculties" fumed the first lady.

The president was gently eased from his stuporous state of sleep. The surgical teams patched the incisions as they removed the life lines. The total volume of blood brought back into his body, the Maquet had performed admirably to keep the seriously jeopardized mission afloat. Now very much on his own as he fought feverishly to restore some semblance of his former chipper self.

After the 'minimally invasive' surgery, deemed a success, was completed, they slowly coaxed the commander in chief back to consciousness. The surgeons nodded allowing a brief broadcast in his compromised condition.

"He's groggy, but coherent." A little light headed

as the blood began to bath his brain, like a frat party or cocktail mixer on capitol hill. On the road to a full recovery, still a slippery slope considering all the extraneous circumstances and mitigating factors surmised the skilled surgical staff. Nevertheless, they knew he was a fighter. A winner who wouldn't give up in the face of insurmountable odds or adversity. 'Winners never quit, quitters never win' he was oft told by a prominent businessman and American icon, Donald Trump. He took the words to heart if only in his dreamy state. It seemed to do the trick, the placebo to hurl him over the edge into the here and now as he came to.

"We'll bring him up to speed" assured the seasoned vet. He'd seen many men literally come back from the dead off the battlefield. This case certainly not much different. Certainly more modern MASH units and methods, yet the will of the warrior a vital tour de force in the awakening and road to recovery. A long road to Tiperary, still a long way to go, before the precious stem cells could differentiate into the vital tissues and regenerate the lost walls.

"Out of the frying pan, into the fire" chuckled Pam. Just when they thought they had put him out of his misery, he was broadsided by a mountain of insurmountable stress. The repair may have been pointless. She figured they'd need to start a tour boat service inside the president's coronary arteries soon. Everyone would soon come onboard the medical break through band wagon.

14: Out of Sight?

'As a rule what is out of sight, generally disturbs men's minds more than what they see.'

- Julius Caeser, Roman general and statesman

"What time is it?" asked Dr Mancini, as they were led into the control center. The Atomic Clock near the top of the midnight hour. Its hands seemed to stand still. A slow steady blip emanated from the prostrate patient's chest cavity on the screen. The little submersible souvenir to leave a lasting impression, possibly forever.

"Much later than we thought" suggested Pam perturbed by the proximity of the hands of the 'doomsday' clock to a final confrontation and countdown; and the menacing problem that now plagued the planet. She checked her watch to synchronize it with the official pace keeper. The medical specialists had kept up their end of the bargain. The onus was now on the naval, air force military and defense department head honchos to keep up theirs. Dragging their butts in an imminent brutal showdown and standoff, that could obliterate everything and everyone from the face of the earth.

"Washington's burning?"

"Brighter than a 4th of July fireworks fiasco…"

"Boy, take some time off and more than our beds are burnin'… burnin' down the house, the White-house that is!" worried Pam. "Just how long were we gone?"

"I was about to suggest that the president in his present condition be subject to as little stress as possible…" insisted Dr Mancini offering his sound medical advice. At the breakthrough news broadcast he placed his chances at slim to nil of a recovery. “So much for preventive medicine.”

**

The rebels raided and ramsacked the respected inner recesses of the Kremlin. They caught most of the politicians off guard, rounding them up then herding them into holding cells.

“I always said we must ‘shrink’ the size of government” stated the riled rebel leader ridiculed for his radical extremist views, he’d finally have his day in the private council chambers to present his particular point of view. As more top political leaders were hurried and shuffled off to remote Bolshevik oblast gulags, Putemkin mulled the origins of the highly orchestrated operation,

“An inside job?” he mused. One of his stunned top advisors concurred.

“It would seem so” he stated as he too was hauled away in shackles. A complete and utter hostile takeover now in progress. Coupled with the sudden counter insurgency activity across the pond, the conditions were slowly coming to a boil. Putemkin was led to the Russian equivalent of the situation room and sated in front of the television cameras to make an official statement of declaration. With a gun to his head, he questioned their intentions and motives for the unacceptable, reprehensible act of violence.

"We're reasonable men unlike our political leaders" laughed the demented despot. Putemkin questioned his sanity without insisting upon a psychiatric exam. The writing and signs clearly on the wall and hallowed halls of the Russian House and senate. "We're not demanding a ransom, we're simply going to send them all up the creek..uh Volga without how do you say?" He turned to his colleague or translator who whispered in his ear, "A paddle." The transmission came through loud and clear on all secure military channels in the US; most restored to some satisfactory degree.

AFI patched them through to the CMDF and Marine One. The president was propped up to capture the compromised position of both seats of power. The White House literally wiped off the map, erased like yesterday's news. The Kremlin capitulated at the hands of likely the same mad men who'd orchestrated the blast. The first of many? The point of origin still unknown, possibly revamped leftovers from the cold war era. Statisticians were working round the clock to come up with answers. The president prompted a weak faint smile as he faced his foes.

"What does that lunatic want?" asked Dr Mancini monitoring president Taylor's vitals closely. His heart skipped a few beats at the mere minute brief he'd received and at the sight of the slovenly attired, disheveled appearance of the terrorist thugs. Dr Mancini eyed the paddles, the cardio resuscitating defibrillators standing by at a moment's notice to jump start his heart if the situation warranted it. He could keel over any second thought the seasoned heart specialist.

"They just don't see the 'big' picture" rambled the rebel leader, his demands as of yet unclear.

"Good God, he plans to reduce them all to Russian raisins. Putemkin a prune?"

The surgeon missed most of the translation focusing on the nutritional benefit to a highly modified diet, low in polyunsatured fats, high in omega three fatty acids, etc and heard only..

"Not a bad idea, along with a bowl of oat bran, or mountain mix of Muesli and 2% milk" he mused and mulled a daily regimen to insure the swiftest course to his chipper former self. The shocking revelation left the Russian rebel spell bound. He then burst into a riveting display of disapproval as he learned of the world's leader's whereabouts.

"What is this, some sort of trick photography?" His fellow henchmen tried to subdue him and bring him from a boil to a slow simmer. They urged him to maintain his cool in front of the television cameras. They'd come this far to secure an uplink and downlink, patching into the very heart of the enemy. They couldn't botch the brilliant takeover attempt! Not NOW! "He's dead! I tell you! Agent Dmitry delivered the knock out punch!"

Still very much alive thanks to the miraculous medical intervention, on two accounts, for it prevented his appearance at the old ball game the previous evening. The president cracked a feisty faint smile and a futile attempt to force a hearty laugh.

"Looks like you miscalculated, you madman!" mentioned the VP from his lofty perch in Marine One. The helicopter wove in and out of the dense smoke soon to touch down. "The president indeed was undergoing a medical exam. And well out of harm's way!" The surgeon called his bluff. Dr Mancini added insult to injury by indicating "He passed with flying colors!" as he opted to let the cameras focus on a strong steady heart beat and vitals. The solid waves, definitely a good sign.

"NOOOOOO!" fumed the confused and flustered fiend. He was stark raving mad at the unexpected turn of events. His plot foiled albeit the collateral damage could reach into the tens of thousands as casualty reports continued to pour into the AFI intercepted frequencies. Not the sort of numbers the president wanted to hear. He'd rather receive their vote of confidence then absentee ballots at the upcoming primaries. The election furthest from his mind at the moment. He had to get a handle on things or there may not be a state senator or country to vote for.

"It looks like our hands are tied Mr President" stated president Taylor as he planned to pitch temporary albeit binding terms to a peace proposal and non proliferation pact. To end the expansion and dissemination of the wretched WMD's once and for all! One for all and all for one was his motto.

"There's always one ….in the crowd. ready to plunge his knife into our backs" stated the steady firm leader in the face of certain death as the demented desperados decided what to do next. The president had certainly thrown a monkey wrench into the madmen's modus operandi.

"Or chest?" chuckled the president, getting back to his irascible resourceful, full of vim, vigor and humorous self.

"Don't just sit there!" snapped the first lady equally shocked to see him up and at 'em so soon. He certainly looked like his former self. A stand in or actor in lieu of certainly a concern for the joint chiefs of staff. "Do something!" she demanded. He hadn't relinquished his command to her or any of their subordinates, not by any stretch of the imagination, other than the miraculous life saving measures completed only moments ago. "Call off the attack!" she urged. The seconds ticked away. A series of irrevocable moves soon initiated irreversibly to alter the course of history forever. The rockets to Russia would soon fill the skies over the Kremlin. Finding their way up the Volga and from every missile base bordering the Russian heartland.

"We're going to give president Putemkin an early retirement, as I'm sure Dmitry had wanted to give you personally" barked the cold blooded Bolshevik killer boldly. He'd stop at nothing, now that he'd gotten this far. Past the point of no return. The thought of spending the rest of his life in a gulag or face the firing squad, unthinkable. There was no turning back now.

"I can't speak for my comrade's retirement plans. I can only tell you about yours" said the president facetiously. Much stronger, able to navigate the nemeses' ways and means. The skilled tactician made it very clear, "The United States does not bargain with terrorists!"

"Our nukes are locked on target sir, including targets just outside Moscow" stated the defense secretary and joint chiefs of staff. The president caught the drift, the pitch unmistakable. To strike swiftly, and knock out the GRU facility, presumably the source of the surprise gift, a Russian flotilla floating up the Potomac. Neither the time nor proper place for its reappearance. He preferred to study the vessels in a Moscow naval museum or some form of figure in a photograph from one of Jane's Fighting Ship's volumes. An aficionado of the land sea and air forces, he oft immersed his mind in the latest greatest military innovations. The JSF 35 Lightning IIs topped that list. Their legendary performance came to the fore again. They'd thwarted an enemy raid up the river right in their own backyard!

"Estimated collateral damage?" questioned the VP of the United States. A display of military might must be initiated before any hostile force gained ground in the scenario. Opt for a stalemate? A stand off? An eye for an eye? Tit for tat? The Russians needed to know America would not let anyone meddle with them. Heavy metal hardware was armed and ready to roll off the decks of several US aircraft carriers in the region. Moscow a few minutes away by air. And if their intelligence sources served them correctly, hit a decided blow below the belt and knock out the secret GRU miniaturization facility! Reputed to reside just outside Moscow. The statisticians ran a few numbers scenarios for the suburb and subdivision of the Russian capitol. They calculated wind and weather patterns, favorable forecast, inclemental conditions. Sufficient firepower to penetrate the perimeter defenses and deliver the deadly dose of and a taste of their own medicine.

"A few thousand innocent GRU agents and scientists" estimated the advanced counter insurgency sources and spies located in Moscow.

"The BI bombers are air born sir." A state of impasse not highly improbable. The fate of the free world now hinged on a conciliatory counter measure. Putemkin had to save face yet swallow the bitter pill. The first strike was delivered by one of their own residents, irrespective of color, cloth or political affiliation. The rebel factions and leader had his day in the privy council chambers. But this is where it would end. It wouldn't get beyond the hallowed halls of either world headquarter. All the terrorists could hope for is buy a little more time as they rounded up a few more politicians and whisked them to the miniaturization facility. Indeed living up to his word to 'shrink the size of government'. The rebels rapidly reduced the wretched ruling class to miniature misfits, then in turn to wisps of the world leaders they once were. Gone for good, washed away like grains of sand, the incredible shrinking machine had done enough dirty work for one day. Not the greater good that the CMDF envisioned. The good, bad and the ugly truth of any new innovative technology soon realized. In the hands of a madman, mindless needless death and destruction. In the hands of the hero, a heart warming welcome and quantum leap and advance in modern medicine.

"Your time's run out mr President!" ribbed the rebel. His poker face neither disarming or particularly persuasive. The president called his bluff and ordered the preemptive strike. He'd face his maker and higher authority one day. He knew the senseless slaughter of thousands a heavy price to pay. Yet to preserve peace and even the playing field, he needed to put an end to the possibility of further illicit use of the technology. Putemkin swallowed his pride in Russian know how. How, where and exactly when the GRU agents had swiped the highly coveted CMDF secrets still a mystery. The why obviously answered in the cunning charade. The shenanigans would go no further. The rebels without a cause would pay for their actions. Putemkin or his successor would see to it should he perish or succumb to the sordid demands of the wretched perpetrators in the disturbing power coupe.

"On the contrary, gentlemen GRU has got to go! Lets give them a taste of their own medicine.

"A bitter pill to swallow" stated the Russian president despondently. He faced his demons and all the demented terrorists demands before. He had to cede to US retaliatory strike, the repercussions impossible to determine. As far as they were all concerned it would be made to look like a catastrophic accident to cause no further alarm or concern. The international incidents, ill time cataclysmic coincidences, both demonstrating the immediate and utterly devastating effects of atoms gone wild! The message would reverberate around the world, loud and clear, WMDs have got to GO! Non proliferation pacts and radical reduction in their manufacture, deployment and use of these deadly deterrents. Decidedly down to nil.

Eradicated off the face of the earth once and for all. There was nothing left to discuss or say. The ramifications and actions spoke infinitely more than mere words or parchments of paper upon which signatures were placed. The time had come to bring about a world peace to insure the sanctity of our species for countless future generations.

"It will look like an accident, an experimental error, agreed?"

Putemkin said a small prayer for the Russian scientists about to be erased from their positions, yet indelibly etched in the memories and minds of their fellow colleagues, families and the history books of the Russian people.

"Agreed. They will be done.... on earth.... An eye for an eye!" The fuming rebels ranted and raved in defiance yet were ultimately powerless to intervene. Putemkin nodded and acknowledged it was the best way in which to carry out swift, sound justice.

"To remove the mote out of our brother's eye God forgive me..."

The launch codes were activated. A squadron of JSF Lightning II fighter jets split and separated from their wing shaped formation, the lead pilot locked on target. A small nuclear tipped cruise missile fell from the belly of the beast then bore down on a quaint university type suburb near Moscow as it broke through some obscured cloud cover. It eluded the Russian defense forces, hit without warning, like white lightning and soon converged on the miniaturization complex.

In the facility the fuming rebel forces flailed about unleashing rounds of ammo from their AK 47's into the air. In a futile last ditch effort to thwart the attack they held their hostages, the unsuspecting GRU agents and scientists at bay. A blessing in disguise for the end would come in the wink of an eye. Not knowing perhaps the best course of action. In a flash it was over. The facility was flattened depressed into a crater like formation no more mystifying than had an asteroid struck the surface of the planet. The shock waves were felt around the earth.

"Good riddance" stated Putemkin. "We'll grow some more" he stated defiantly not to be out done by his American counterpart. He'd insure the riff and chaff were weeded out this time in the highly innovative home grown remedy. Likely learn a few tips from the aspiring medical specialists and president Taylor himself one day in the near future. he hoped they could mend their bruised egos and affairs of the heart in a timely fashion. The chilling chapter in world political history slowly drew to a close. The president made a rapid recovery.

"Looks like the president is back to his irascible self" as he prepared to give the state address. There was so much work to do to rebuild the capitol bigger and better than ever before. The Kremlin too suffered a crushing blow as it was radically 'shrunk' in size.

"When life throws you Yemens, you make Yemenade!" quipped the thought provoking leader of the free world. The source of the briefcase nuke was traced back to a terrorist safe house in Aden, the Yemeni capitol. Teams of tactical undercover CIA agents and navy seals planned a surprise visit of their own. Justice delivered swiftly and concertedly.

"Thank God, I'll live to see another day. So will our families and countless future generations" he stated appreciatively. His heart pounding rapidly at the sight of the swift reparations already underway in DC. His heart leapt a few beats. Heart burn or merely indigestion? His new low calorie diet and physical fitness routine attributable to his speedy recovery and complete rejuvenation. He often wondered what had happened to the unsung hero, Sam - Sub Atomic Man to a few close colleagues. He'd remain forever indelibly etched in their hearts and minds. Perhaps it was he who given his life for him and the ill fated albeit successful mission? He shook his head in wonder.

Inside the cavernous spaces of his heart, the totipotent cardiac stem cells had sprouted and grown to full maturity matching the former myocardium free from atherosclerotic plague and occluded dead heart muscle. The thriving red blood cells flourished and infiltrated the furrows, now hardly recognizable in the rapid transformation. The only growing concern, one errant piece of carry on luggage left on board the Proteus that day, long since swallowed up by the body's defense mechanism. The shiny briefcase lodged in the wall of the heart, either overlooked by the macrophages or somehow recognized as self, outstanding in the field for so long like a feisty ferocious scarecrow. The small nuclear device literally like a ticking time bomb about to go off at any second continued to send a faint signal like a transponder from a satellite sent to a distant galaxy. This signal from inner space no less baffling. One day, the recipients to receive the message loud and clear? The clear and present danger inside the president's pericardium persisted to this very day. Where and when the next heart flutter or palpitation would occur, setting off an irreversible sequence of events, was anyone's guess. It might be wise to pay a visit to his heart specialist once in a while. The sooner the better, before the problem may be blown out of proportion again. Dr Mancini agreed and scheduled a return visit to the scene of the spectacular stem cell staged performance. A newer Proteus was reconstructed form the initial designs. Modified with a few updated features and so forth. Better to be safe than sorry figured the renown heart specialist.

The president lapsed into a state of suspended animation. Still a little light headed, side effects from the blood perfusion? He wondered if he'd dreamt the entire far fetched episode.

"How long was I under? Did I miss anything?" His steel claw trap memory needed a refresher course to recall the roster of political replacements or simply the first sign of forgetfulness, heaven forbid senility.

"No dear, you were just doing your job, playing world leader…" reassured the first lady. Stories to relive by the campfire, for future generations captivated by the tall tale, no more miraculous or unbelievable than Paul Bunyan and the giant Blue Ox 'Babe', only diametrically opposed on opposite ends of the size spectrum, yet no less fascinating, spirited or far fetched.

President Taylor and President Putemkin gathered and met once again on a more peaceful note at the signing of the Washington-Moscow Nuclear Non Proliferation Treaty in Washington. Repairs were well underway. The reminders like those of Chernobyl still indelibly etched into the landscape.

"Today marks a historic date for mankind where we can assure a world free of weapons of mass destruction…"

"So our children and grand children can live in peace free from the threat of global mutual annihilation" stated Putemkin.

A 21gun salute resonated through the respected sacred memorial grounds. Sam was honored with a hero's sound off & medal of honor posthumously.

A couple children launched their toy boats along the shore of Hampton Roads, near the site of the Monitor and Merrimack standoff oblivious of what had taken place only a few short months ago.

EPILOGUE

SAM, Sub Atomic Man was never seen or heard from ever again. The incredible shrinking man disappeared into oblivion, yet through his memorable life saving methods, he salvaged the entire crew of the tiny submersible Proteus. Lost to the president's remarkable immunological defense system. Rebuilt better and stronger than before, the question remained, would the body recognize its replacement? The newer prototype sat silently on the launch pad awaiting its next crew and orders to initiate the next death defying stunt or surgical mission. Named the Nautilus in honor of Captain Nemo's vessel. Bound to go where no man had gone before. 20,000 leagues under the sea or through the circulatory system in the inner personal private space of the next patient. It might as well be 20,000 light years into outer space, either adventure equally as compelling and challenging.

https://www.cdc.gov/heart-disease/data-research/facts-stats/index.html

https://pmc.ncbi.nlm.nih.gov/articles/PMC8788183/

https://www.sciencedirect.com/topics/medicine-and-dentistry/cardiac-stem-cell

https://pmc.ncbi.nlm.nih.gov/articles/PMC4208604/

Devlin, Kate. British Doctors Help Perform the World's First Transplant of a Whole Organ grown in a lab. Nov 18, 2008. Telegraph. UK.

First Human receives Cardiac Stem Cells in Clinical Trial to Heal Heart Damage caused by Heart Attack. July 1, 2009. Medical News Today.

https://en.wikipedia.org/wiki/Endogenous_cardiac_stem_cell

Maquet HL 20 Machine. www.maquet.com

Asimov, Isaac. Fantastic Voyage. Bantam Books. NY. 1966.

Drexler, K. Eric. 'Father of Nanotechnology'. Founder Foresight Institute. www.e-drexler.com

Fuller, Buckminster 'Bucky'. Thinking Out Loud. PBS 'American Masters' TV documentary on the inventor, visionary, thinker.(lecture Uof C c1978)

Sub Atomic Man (SAM) has the 'metagene', found in humans that have the ability to develop super human powers and based loosely on:

Atom, DC Comics superhero Ray Palmer named after former science fiction magazine editor; makes a lens from white dwarf matter to shrink to subatomic size

Captain Atom: DC version of Nathaniel Adam, air force pilot, 'atomized' in experimental nuclear blast; his love interest Dr Angela Spica, PhD physicist, 'Engineer', 'The Maker', infused with blood nanites that can shape change, transform

Ant Man, Marvel Comic Superhero-Dr Henry Pym discovers 'Pym's Particles', shrinking ability

Lunev, Stanislav. Through the Eyes of the Enemy: The Autobiography of Stanislav Lunev. Regnery Publishing, Washington. DC. 1998. (Russian GRU defector, re: missing Russian 'suitcase' nukes)

DC Crater: Fact or Fiction? Crater Hypothesis 35 million years ago. Traces of Catastrophe. Pg 105 8.7. Impacts and the early earth. French, B.M.

Woolf, Amy. Specialist in Nuclear Policy. Non Strategic Nuclear Weapons. Congressional Research Service. Aug. 10, 2009.

The Raw Story. CNN: Mystery 9/11 aircraft was military 'doomsday plane'. Sept 13, 2007.

Boeing E-4 Advanced Airborn Command Post, Project 'Nightwatch'

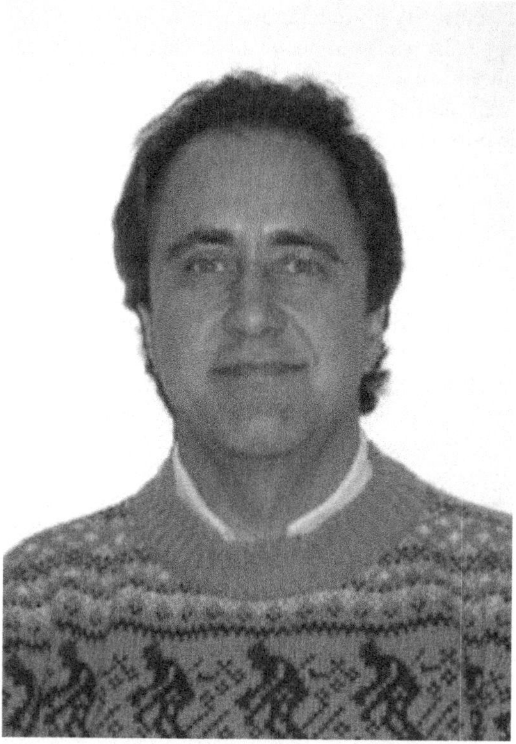

The author, Bernie Unrau, an implant dentist by training, stumbled across a four minute video back in 1989, an interview with the prolific Robin Cook, a physician by training. His mastery of the medical thriller inspired Bernie to embark on a 2nd career and a new uncharted course each summer. The central character in his novels, Dr Gum, perhaps part bumbling lieutenant Columbo or the deductive Sherlock Holmes the imaginary detective created by Sir Conan Doyle, also a physician; the tenacity of Dr Ryan conceived by Tom Clancy, or the curiosity of Indiana Jones A dash of the dapper James Bond blended in, shaken and stirred into the equation the inspiration of in depth concept research of Michael Crichton and his creations or the powerful suspense of a John Grisham legalistic thriller. Or to simply bring some of his years as a dentist, lecturer and inventor to light by engaging in espionage, elucidating an enigma, disclosing the dastardly or diabolical scheme, or dreaming up a formidable frightening future. And as the prolific Zane Grey, dentist turned novelist turned screen-writer, pen 100 books. The author has enjoyed travel, tennis, sailing, skiing, flying, reading and thinking. He is single and currently resides in Calgary, Alberta.

Books by Dr Bernie Unrau:

Terra Vista
Deadly Implant
Not A Drop
Golden Mask
Questa
Rook
Hooked
Big B
Enlightened
The Board
The ROM
New Millenium
Reflections
Submarine Slide
Sabotage
Dentinator
Ubar
Stemwinder
Pulling Strings
Meltdown
Pulpit Fiction
Confusion
Glazers
God Almighty
The Scrying
Rising
Cravings
Fantastic Voyage III
East of Aden
The X Files: The Grey Zone
Lacryma Christi
In Gold We Trust
Lion Island
Dead Hand

Dream Big
The Fifth Pillar
Blowout
The Six Billion Dollar Man
The Hearsemen
The Substantiator
Ultra Stealth: War Games
Alien Vengeance
Finger of God
Justice League Doomed
You Can't Tek It With You
Switchblade
Now You See Me 3
The Great Museum Heist
Pirates of the Deep Web
Ezekiel's Wheel
Raid
Bury Me Under The Volvano
Bond Jane Bond
Deep Fright
The Bang Bang Boys
Bloody Mary
Winner
Catch Me When You Can
Phantom of the Operatory
Zombie Street
Bad to the Bone
Jabberwhacky
Sweet Tooth
Subterranea
Pandemonium
Trillions
Apes and Aliens
The Privateers
Not Yet
Kick Ass Kasino

Deep Fright Down Under
Deep Fright Deep Freeze
Curse of the Seven Pagodas
Chokepoint
The Ice Forest
Power Heist
Chinatown Tequila
Alien Vengeance: Raising Cain
Goldfield
The Mansion of Dr M
Ticking Time Bomg
Quicksilver
Big Fat Liars
Mother of Pearl
Route 666
Game Over
Montauk Monster
Guardians of the Genome
The Floathouse
Alpha and Omega
Nightwalker
Insight
The Glass
The Narrow Gate
The Sleep Committee
Venus Grotto
Catch 22
Mind at Large
Spearphish
Salt Shaker
Prodigy the New Frontier
Fantastic Voyage
Terror Island
Titanpointe

Screenplays by Dr Bernie Unrau:

Terra Vista
Deadly Implant
Not A Drop
Golden Mask
Questa
Rook
Hooked
Big B
Enlightened
The Board
The ROM
New Millenium
Reflections
Submarine Slide
Sabotage
Dentinator
Ubar
Stemwinder
Pulling Strings
Meltdown
Pulpit Fiction
Confusion
Glazers
God Almighty
The Scrying
Rising
Fantastic Voyage III
East of Aden
Cravings
The X Files: the Grey Zone
Chokepoint
Ultra Stealth: War Game
Phantom of the Operatory

Montauk Monster
Deep Fright
Jabberwhacky
Pandemonium
Deep Fright: Down Under
The Curse of the 7 Pagodas
Sweet Tooth
The Ice Forest
The Frozen Chosen
Insight
Subterranea
The Glass
Deep Fright: Deep Freeze
Sky Parlor
The Movie Mobile
Nightwalker
Venus' Grotto
Big Fat Liar 2
The Space Bar
Spearphish
Mind At Large
Summa Gate
Not Yet
Finger of God
Terror Island
Game Over
Salt II
Death Valley Riders
Apes & Aliens
Zombie Street
Catch Me When You Can
Bloody Mary
Raid
Bury Me Under The Volcano
The Privateers
Bond Jane Bond

You Can't Take It With You
Catch 22
The Float House
Alien Vengeance
Alien Vengeance: Raising Cain
The Great Museum Heist
Magic is in the Hare
Goldfield
Quicksilver
Bad to the Bone
In Gold We Trust
Lion Island
Dead Hand
The Fifth Pillar

Made in the USA
Monee, IL
04 November 2026

67385526R00164